The Early History of Surgery in Great Britain

Also from Westphalia Press
westphaliapress.org

The Early History of Surgery in Great Britain

Its Organization and Development

by G. Parker,
M.A., M.D., M.R.C.S.

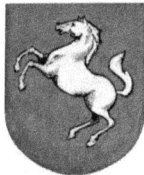

WESTPHALIA PRESS
An imprint of Policy Studies Organization

Westphalia Press
An imprint of Policy Studies Organization
1527 New Hampshire Ave., NW
Washington, D.C. 20036
info@ipsonet.org

ISBN-13: 978-1-63391-381-3
ISBN-10: 1-63391-381-3

Cover design by Taillefer Long at Illuminated Stories:
www.illuminatedstories.com

Daniel Gutierrez-Sandoval, Executive Director
PSO and Westphalia Press

Updated material and comments on this edition
can be found at the Westphalia Press website:
www.westphaliapress.org

THE EARLY HISTORY
OF SURGERY
IN GREAT BRITAIN

ITS ORGANIZATION AND DEVELOPMENT

BY

G. PARKER, M.A., M.D., M.R.C.S.
MAJOR R.A.M.C.(T.)

A. & C. BLACK, LTD.
4, 5 & 6 SOHO SQUARE, LONDON, W.C. 1
1920

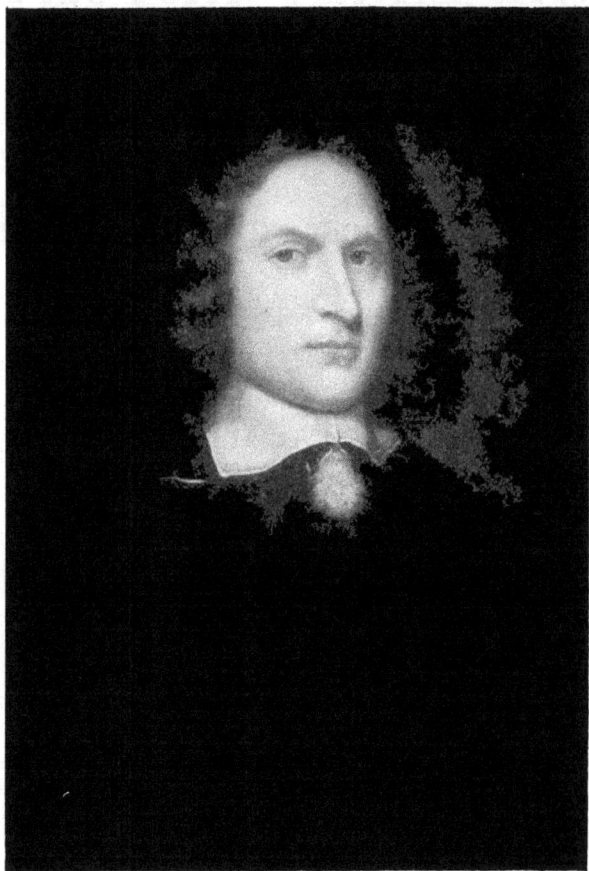

RICHARD WISEMAN,

SERGEANT SURGEON TO CHARLES II.

Autotype from an oil-painting in the possession of the Royal College of Surgeons.

PREFACE

In the following pages I have tried to trace in detail the revival and early surroundings of the surgical art after the end of the dark ages of Europe, and to point out the social movements which influenced its progress.

I had been investigating for some time various questions connected with the ancient therapeutic gilds in this country—which, by the way, turned out to be largely surgical—when the opportunity was offered me of giving in this short volume some account of the early history of surgery. This would of necessity include the effects of these bodies, and of other social and political institutions, on the organization of surgery and the education of students. I hope that I have not been led to allot too much space to this part of my subject, and that other important matters— such as the influence of the three great scientific revivals in Europe and of the lives and work of the chief surgeons of each period—have been clearly though briefly described.

I am well aware of the errors which, in spite of every care, must occur in an attempt to give an outline of so many centuries in so short a space; if I have not found it possible to insert in the text my authority for every statement, and always to acknowledge my indebtedness to other writers, I have at least given a list of the authorities at the end, which will also be useful to students.

I have to thank Dr. R. Shingleton Smith and other friends for helping me with the proofs, Dr. Freeland Fergus, President of the Royal Faculty in Glasgow, the Barbers' Company in London, the Corporation of Bristol, Mr. Henry S. Wellcome, Sir D'Arcy Power, and Dr. J. D. Comrie, for the loan of beautiful illustrations.

G. P.

CONTENTS

CHAPTER I

1000 TO 1300 A.D.

CHAPTER II

1300 TO 1500 A.D.

CHAPTER III

1500 TO 1600 A.D.

CHAPTER IV

1600 TO 1700 A.D.

CHAPTER V

1700 TO 1800 A.D.

CHAPTER VI

1800 TO 1850 A.D.

LIST OF ILLUSTRATIONS

THE
EARLY HISTORY OF SURGERY
IN BRITAIN

CHAPTER I

1000 TO 1300 A.D.

1. GENERAL SURVEY OF THE TIMES

IN a discussion on the growth of any art in a given
country we have first to settle at what date we
shall begin. Now we do not propose to spend
time in discussing the surgical knowledge of the
Roman rulers of Britain, for classical medicine and
surgery has been already elucidated, but even that
would not take us to the beginning of the art.
There were heroes before Agamemnon and surgeons
among neolithic men. Our knowledge of the past
was, until lately, bounded strictly by Roman,
Greek, and Hebrew civilizations, but during the
life of the present generation the curtain has been
lifted, and we have minute knowledge of the social
life of immense periods in many places. Egyptian,
Ægean, Assyrian, and some prehistoric civiliza-

1

tions are unfolding their medical and surgical knowledge. Thus, ere long we may be expected to describe the surgery of the Lake Dwellers in England and that of the Norse Vikings, who, we are now told, were highly civilized country gentlemen with a trifle of the political ideas of the modern Germans. Indeed, there are plenty of facts already showing the surgical skill of many primitive races, such as the Australians and prehistoric Egyptians, and something may be gleaned as to the earliest dwellers in Britain, but this we shall also omit.

The surgical knowledge, again, in the warring states of Britain during Anglo-Saxon times seems to us singularly small. Perhaps this is due to our ignorance. One would have thought that many remnants of knowledge from older civilizations would have survived in one or more of the many races which make up the extraordinarily mixed nationality to which we belong. But the Africo-Iberian, Celtic, German, and Scandinavian settlers, not to mention the descendants of the Roman officials and Greek traders, seem to have retained very few fragments of ancient learning. The ability was there, as we see in the wonderful outburst of literature which followed the introduction of Christianity, but the accumulated stores of medical knowledge had gone. Even the efforts of a few teachers from Constantinople and Rome had little effect on the general ignorance. Indeed, the whole of Western Europe was in much the same condition, showing how easily great and settled states of civilization may vanish from the earth. We may be told that this view of early Britain is too narrow, and be reminded of Celtic hereditary physicians, of the monasteries, of the Saxon leech books, and the stories of surgical work preserved in the lives of Hilda, Frideswide, and others.

However, in the scanty space we have, it seem better here to omit altogether half the years which separate us from the Roman Conquest, interesting as they are, and to commence our task with the second half—*i.e.*, about the year A.D. 1000. Even then in the first parts of our story we shall find the materials are scanty, but thanks to the labours of Freind and in recent days of Payne, Norman Moore, D'Arcy Power, and others, we are learning that there are facts to be gleaned; and it is probable that they will be greatly multiplied. For though the documents directly relating to surgery are extremely few for the earliest periods, the general historical records in this country are more abundant than anywhere else. As they are opened up fresh and unexpected light is being thrown on technical subjects. That great activity and interest in surgery and medicine existed in early times is clear from the enormous development of hospitals at one period, and of anatomical research at another, from the medical libraries, such as the 500 volumes at Canterbury about 1500, from the military organization of surgeons, and from the elaborate teaching system of the barber surgeons in various towns.

Nor were the methods and aims of ancient writers so absurd as the casual reader may imagine. Their quaint phraseology and the absurd theories they put forward to explain their facts, and indeed our habit of selecting ludicrous passages for quotation, are apt to blind us to their work and meaning, and to the identity of their aims with ours in a given operation, for example.   In many instances the very methods we have adopted were discovered by them, and then disused and forgotten.   Posterity will equally laugh over our technical language, and the theories brought forward in the scientific papers of to-day, when the style has faded with time.

The development of surgery in this country, it will be seen, falls into four periods or stages. First, that which followed the sudden appearance of universities and hospitals in Europe in the twelfth century.   *Second,* that due to the great Renaissance and the elaborate educational system of the barber surgeons in the sixteenth century.   *Third,* that which sprang from the revival of hospitals and

commencement of hospital schools and clinical
teaching in the eighteenth century ; and, *lastly*,
the present period which anæsthetics and the discoveries of Pasteur and Lister have made possible.
This last stage will not be discussed in these pages.

2. THE GROWTH OF SURGERY ABROAD AND AT HOME FROM 1000 TO 1300

In this period surgery began to show the first signs
of revival after the ruin of European civilization by
the Barbarians. It did more, for towards 1300
a great and rapid development took place, first
in the Italian universities and then among the
practitioners of surgery everywhere. Besides the
contributions of contemporary surgeons, two
streams of knowledge came to Europe. In the
Eastern Empire classical medicine had survived
and produced such teachers as Alexander of Tralles
and Paul of Ægina, while the Arabist school had
joined to their knowledge of Greek medicine
the discoveries of Rhazes, Avicenna, and Albucasis.
The teaching of these two schools reached us in
the following ways: (1) At Monte Cassino, the
first Benedictine monastery, the study of medicine
had begun as early as 850, and a hospital was
founded by Abbot Desiderius in 1050. Here
Constantinus, the African who gave the name
variola to smallpox, translated for Europe some of

the Arabist writings, with at least one surgical treatise. (2) In the twelfth century Gerard of Cremona translated Albucasis, whose work became the chief surgical textbook for the Italian universities, and was itself derived through Paul of Ægina from Celsus and Galen. (3) The Medical School at Salerno, near Naples (800-1250), also got access both to the writings of the classical and the Arabist authors, and gave special study to the practical side of medicine, the symptoms of disease, anatomy, and the principles of dietetics and pharmacy. Students were obliged to devote seven years to their work and pass an examination in Hippocrates, Galen, and the Arabists. Among the writings of this school the *Compendium*, an encyclopædia of medicine by six authors, and the *Regimen Sanitatis Salerni*, a popular rhyming treatise on the rules of health, are frequently referred to, and an unnamed textbook which was translated into Anglo-Saxon for English use. The two first great surgeons of mediæval Europe, Roger (1180) and Roland (1250), appeared here, besides Copho, the anatomist, and several women doctors. Roger's *Practice of Surgery* shows him able to employ sutures and ligatures for bleeding, but favouring suppuration by dressing with ointments. *The Glosses of the Four Masters*, a later amplification of his textbook, attributed the decadence of surgery to two causes—the neglect of anatomy and the separation of medicine and surgery, of which more must be said here later on.

We may now turn from these early efforts to consider the vigorous growth of surgery in the Italian universities of the thirteenth century, that early Renaissance when mediæval science, art, political thought reached their most brilliant stage. Cultivated and really able surgeons taught students from every part of Europe, and a remarkable movement for surgical reform took place, which was no less than an anticipation of Lister's teaching —viz., extreme cleanliness and the abolition of all the cumbrous ointments and dressings of the past, except lint soaked in alcohol or wine, with a view to obtain primary union of wounds. The leaders of this movement were first :

Theodoric (1205-1295) of Bologna, who has been called one of the most original surgeons of any age. He was Bishop of Cervia and a pupil of Hugh of Lucca. His great treatise on surgery appeared in 1266, and it is noteworthy that the account of leprosy in it was taken from an English writer, Gilbert. He became the pioneer of the new teaching, and lays down that "it is not necessary, as modern surgeons teach, that pus should be generated in wounds. No error can be greater than this. Such a practice hinders nature and prevents the agglutination of the wound " (Clifford Allbutt, *Historical Relations of Medicine and Surgery*). He rejected the use of ointments and salves, washed the wound with wine only, removing every trace of foreign bodies, brought the edges together as dry and clean as possible, and laid on it lint steeped in wine to evaporate. In old wounds he refreshed the edges after thorough cleansing, so that the natural exudation might unite them. His teaching was adopted by Arnold, of Villanova, who used the newly discovered spirits of wine or alcohol, and his work was carried on in its essentials, though with some modifications, by Salicet, Lanfranc, and Mondeville.

William Salicet (1201-1277), a military surgeon educated in the University of Bologna, where he became city physician, investigated the causes of healing by first intention, and wrote a standard treatise on surgery based on his own case histories. He was able to suture divided nerves and to diagnose arterial bleeding from venous. To him we owe the first description of dropsy due to kidney disease, and the restoration of the use of the knife in place of the cautery which the Arabist school had favoured.

Lanfranc of Milan, his pupil, another protester against the division of surgery from medicine, and an excellent clinical teacher, wrote the *Chirurgia*

Magna, with the first clear account of concussion of the brain and a brilliant description of the symptoms of fracture of the skull. He was driven from Milan by the Visconti and went to Paris in 1295, and joining the College of St. Côme, became one of the founders of French surgery.

Yperman of Ypres studied under him at Paris, and, returning to the Netherlands, spread the doctrines of the school, and especially the treatment of certain hæmorrhages by ligature and torsion of the arteries.

Jean Pitard, probably another refugee from an Italian university, became surgeon to Philip the Fair and St. Louis. He, too, preached energetically the doctrine of cleanliness and spirit dressings, but his chief fame was the share he took in founding the College of St. Côme at Paris as a new home for surgery.

Henri de Mondeville (1260-1320), the most brilliant of the group, a witty and charming Frenchman, a pupil of Theodoric in Italy, and educated, too, at Montpellier, joined Pitard and Lanfranc at Paris. Clifford Allbutt calls him the last champion in his day of two causes, the solidarity of medicine and surgery, and of union by first intention as opposed to the salve surgery of Galen.

He says there are many more surgeons who know how to cause suppuration than to heal a wound.

Too much faith in books, he adds in another place, chokes natural talent, but education is needed because surgery is not a rude handicraft. He is remembered, too, for his warnings to students, such as: There are certain rich patients who prefer to suffer in body rather than in their purses; and, again: Never dine with a patient who owes you a debt; get your dinner at an inn, or he will find means to deduct his hospitality from your fees. Allbutt tells us that his teaching was to wash the wound scrupulously clean from all foreign matter, to use no probes or tents, except in special circumstances, to apply no oily or irritant dressings, and to avoid the formation of pus, as being not a stage of healing, but a complication.

"When your dressings have been carefully applied, do not interfere with them for some days; keep the air out, for a wound left in contact with air suppurates. However, should pain and heat arise, open and wash out again, or even a poultice may be necessary, but do not pull your dressings about [too often]; nature works better left alone. Beware that your needles are clean, or they will infect the wound. Do not allow the wound to bleed. For oozing use styptics, for jets of blood the cautery, but the disadvantage is that, when the eschar falls off, bleeding may recur. Digital compression for an hour is useful, and acupressure for large vessels, or if the vessel can be isolated let it be drawn out, twisted, and ligatured."

He complains of the furious opposition and abuse which was poured on him by surgeons and laymen when he introduced the method of cleanliness and spirit lotions into France, "so that, had we not been strong in the faith and of repute with the King and the Princes, and also ourselves men of some little learning, we should have had to give up that method." For a time he was successful, and bid fair to antedate the reforms of Lister by nearly 700 years, but his successors fell away in the search for applications which would heal a foul wound directly—*i.e.*, for antiseptics—which the science of the time could not provide. The filthy war wounds, such as those of the Flemish Plain, then, as now, taxed the skill of the surgeon and led to the disappearance of the aseptic method.

We have dwelt at some length on these teachers as showing the able men who practised surgery at this time, and as some indication of the knowledge and skill existing in the medical schools.

3. THE UNIVERSITIES

The great revival and progress of surgery in the Middle Ages in Europe, then, was largely due to the new universities. One of the most striking achievements of the age was the foundation of these bodies, and the enthusiasm for learning which accompanied it.   From henceforth mediæval society contained a numerous class of educated thinkers, in addition to the soldiers, priests, monks, and peasants of the past.   The universities began in various towns as simple craft gilds of students or teachers, which sprang up as "one result of the instinct of association which swept like a wave over the towns of Europe in the eleventh and twelfth centuries" (Rashdall, *Universities of Europe in the Middle Ages*).   They quickly became extraordinarily popular, and the highways were thronged with crowds of poor boys who struggled to those places where a number of masters were to be found who would impart the higher branches of education to students from any country of Christendom.   Such a place was called a *Studium Generale*, and later on some of them, by papal or imperial decree, or by long custom, gave their *magistri* the right afterwards to teach anywhere else where they might go.

Except for Salerno, which stands on a different footing, the earliest of these institutions were Bologna and Paris, both beginning about 1180. Upon one or other of these were modelled the universities which sprang up in all the great districts of Europe to the number of sixty or eighty.   The term university itself originally meant any gild or corporation, and was applied

to the gild of students in the Bologna type of
institution, and to the gild of masters in the
Parisian one, but in the fifteenth century it became
synonymous with *Studium Generale.*

One result of the movement was that physicians
came to be regarded as members of a learned
profession, and where surgery was not divided from
medicine, as in the early Italian universities, surgery
shared in the elevation. It was here that much of
the revival and progress of surgery found its home,
and here the great masters, Theodoric, Lanfranc,
Salicet, and Mondeville, were trained. In Bologna,
about 1260, a scientific school of medicine began
teaching medicine and surgery as well as logic and
grammar, and in its statutes copying the rules of the
gild of law students, who were the original body at
Bologna. The teaching was based on the Arabists,
but anatomy was at once made a subject of study.
Galen, Hippocrates, Avicenna, Averroes, and the
surgery of Brunus were read. There were doctors
of surgery as well as of medicine. The study of
surgery was well organized, too, at Padua, Florence,
Montpellier, and many of the French universities.
On the other hand, in Paris surgeons were excluded
from the university for a long period, and the practice of the art held to be degrading for a scholar.
Where the influence of Paris extended this hindrance to the growth of surgery was felt. "Sur-

geons reared in base apprenticeships, not only illiterate, but forbidden even the means of learning, lay under heavy disadvantages " (Clifford Allbutt).

To some extent this was minimized by the work of the great College of St. Côme, already mentioned, and the brilliant surgeons it turned out. England itself was affected by this folly, as Oxford was probably an offshoot from Paris ; but Paris did not altogether dominate English custom, even when under English rule. As soon as the records of English universities appear, we find surgeons among the graduates ; for instance, Magister Rogerus, cirurgicus, is found giving evidence for the University of Oxford at a coroner's inquest in 1302, and at Southwark there is a Magister Johannes, cirurgicus, in 1312, as well as Magister Petrus, the King's surgeon about 1315. At Oxford the title Magister would hardly be given to a man because he was warden of a gild, but only to a graduate. Licences, too, for the practice of surgery were after a time granted by English universities, but at first, it must be allowed, they did little for the progress of the art. However, before 1300 students from Britain could and did get instruction freely at the universities of Bologna, Montpellier, Padua, Messina, Naples, Sienna, Salamanca, Piacenza, and Seville.

4. THE SEPARATION OF MEDICINE AND SURGERY

In the Middle Ages we are struck with the fact that most physicians came to abstain altogether from surgery, and had no knowledge of it, while the surgeons were equally shut out from medical knowledge and practice. This had not been the case in Hippocratic days. The result now was disastrous. Medicine, without the guidance of surgery, anatomy, chemistry, or the microscope, became a mass of unproved theories, and surgery a rule of thumb for ignorant craftsmen. Progress in either art was almost impossible.

To-day, though the division still exists, in some degree every practitioner is compelled to gain in his student days a working knowledge of both. The mediæval practitioner could not plead the physical impossibility of getting a thorough knowledge of both, for the actual facts known were comparatively few; but at the present time the surgical specialist, for instance, is unable to keep abreast with all the enormous number of discoveries in medicine, bacteriology, and pathology, as well as those in his own art, though he is helpless without their aid. The result is the rapid development of so-called "team work," or the co-operation of various specialists in all important cases. Half a century ago the general practitioner represented a fairly complete union of

medicine and surgery, but separation into specialties
now tends to be necessary, and every reformer has
to devise some plan which will reduce the huge cost
of combined action by various specialists and
prevent the family doctor from sinking into a mere
guide-post to the specialists required. The position
is most serious, but entirely different to that which
led to the mediæval division.

To return to our history, the cause of the
separation has been much debated. Even in Roman
times we find the physicians showing a preference
for speculation over experimental research, and the
mediæval habit of thought was entirely in the same
direction. It relied on logical argument as the
means of arriving at truth, or on the dicta of great
teachers without testing them by examining what
the actual facts in nature are. Hence the high
place they gave to literary studies as compared
with experiment. The teaching and practical work
of Hippocrates and his followers might have
corrected this, but it had only come down to them
in a very fragmentary form, and the Arabist school
about A.D. 1000 had inculcated an abhorrence and
neglect of surgery. Indeed, Chauliac dates the
separation actually from the time of Albucasis.
Again, it has been said that the age was an
aristocratic one, and looked down on any labour of
the hands and those who practised it. Hence

medicine rather than surgery was the profession for a gentleman.

The Western Church, too, has been credited with a large share in producing the division by forbidding all ecclesiastics from teaching or practising surgery.

Now, though religious feelings from early times had protested against the services of priests who shed human blood in war or even by accident, the definite rules of the Church as to surgery do not appear until after the fashion of the times had restricted surgery in some parts of Europe to men of low social standing. They followed rather than created the fashion.

The Lateran Council of 1139 and the Council of Tours, 1163, are constantly quoted on the other side, but, strange to say, *they have not a word about surgery, or the shedding of blood*, though they forbid monks to desert their own monasteries for the study of secular law, medicine, or pharmacy (Canon 9 of the former and Canon 8 of the latter). Indeed, there are plenty of regulations elsewhere ordering priests and monks to attend to their own duties and to abstain from getting money in other occupations. The first definite rule as to surgery which I have discovered is a Decretal of 1216, which forbade priests to act as judges in capital criminal cases, or to serve in certain military forces, and finally interdicted priests, deacons, and subdeacons from

2

practising surgery. But this is two or three centuries after the separation took place, and even the importance of this is not great, for exemptions were freely granted, as in the notable case of Guy de Chauliac, himself a priest and canon.

Indeed, the Decretal would not affect in any degree the university student or a large section of monks, both of whom were in minor orders only. The separation, too, of medicine and surgery hardly existed in Italy or the South of France, under the very eye of the Papal Curia, at least till a very late period. The Council of Bezières, 1310, is an instance of the recognition of the practice of surgery by priests and monks if under proper episcopal licence.

Whatever was the cause, the absurd and fatal division hindered the growth of both medicine and surgery in Western Europe from about A.D. 1100 onwards.

It is most necessary to remember that these great changes in European surgery affected surgery in England almost as much as elsewhere, since from the time of the Norman Conquest and the Crusades this country had become part of the European Commonwealth, and constant intercourse and travel was going on. The Crusades, as military expeditions to places where Greek and Arabist civilizations still survived, assisted to spread know-

ledge of the old systems everywhere, and in the
second place they caused a demand for military
surgeons to accompany the nobles and warriors
who went from every part of Britain and the
Continent to Greece, Egypt, and Palestine.

5. English Physicians and Surgeons

In this period the names of great English
surgeons and physicians are few indeed, and of
their work there are still fewer detailed records.
Dr. Gilbert Maminot and *Dr. Nigel* served under
William the Conqueror.   The latter was rewarded
for his services as a military surgeon with land in
Wiltshire, Hants, and Worcestershire, where, according to Domesday, he held a hide in Droitwich
of the land of St. Guthlac and also Dunclent.   For
a time he was attached to the army of Roger of
Montgomery and other leaders in the campaign on
the Welsh border, but left no writings.   *Bernard
Gordon*, who was probably a Scotsman, went to
Montpellier, and while there wrote the *Lilium
Medicinæ* about 1300, a typical Arabist textbook.
He gives the first account of the modern form of
truss—brachiale ferreum cum lingula ad modum
semicirculi et paratum sicut oportet, and also of
spectacles—which seem to have been invented by
Salvino de Armati about twenty years earlier
(Garrison, *History of Medicine*).   He also wrote the

out for three hundred years, and in 1276 Cairo witnessed the foundation of the huge Al Mansur Hospital, with its noble courts and splashing fountains and convalescent homes, supported on a revenue of £25,000 a year.

In other ages, of course, hospitals had been built. The ancient world had its Asclepia, the Christians of the fourth century raised great institutions at Constantinople, Edessa, and Ephesus of importance in the history of medicine. Hospitals, too, sprang up some three hundred years later at Rome, Lyons, and Paris, where the Hôtel Dieu appeared in 650. The Benedictine and other orders founded fresh ones in the ninth century, but none of these movements compared in force and extent with the marvellous undertakings of the thirteenth and fourteenth centuries. Many institutions then raised were, of course, only almshouses, refuges for the poor and infirm, and travellers' rests, like St. Cross at Winchester, but a proportion of the 750 "hospitia" built in England alone were for the sole treatment of the sick. There were, in addition, many monasteries which maintained hospitals for the sick as well as infirmaria within their walls for their own members. In 1198 Pope Innocent III., being deeply impressed with the efforts made, and longing that still more should be done for the sick, started a fresh crusade to found the

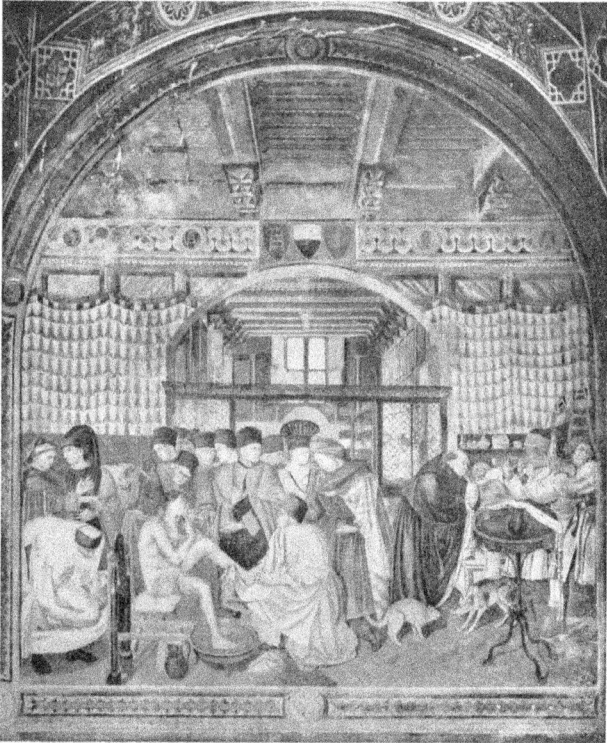

MEDIÆVAL HOSPITAL AT SIENA.

From a fresco by Bartolo.

Hospitals of the Holy Spirit in all the great towns of Europe. Putting himself at the head of the movement, he built at Rome the house of the Santo Spirito in Sassia which still exists. Nine other hospitals were founded at Rome itself, and all over Europe Hospitals of the Holy Spirit sprang up. Virchow reckoned 155 in Germany alone. In many instances these hospitals quickly became municipal institutions, and passed under lay management and control, affording ample opportunities for study to the surgeons and physicians of the towns. Four houses with this dedication existed in England—at Canterbury, Warwick, Hereford, and Taunton—but details of the English houses are obscure and scanty. The nursing was not left to chance. Societies for the purpose were also numerous. The Alexians, the Beguins, the sisters of St. Elizabeth, the brothers of the Holy Ghost, who were laymen, and the hospitallers of St. John were some of these groups of workers.

Where universities and medical schools existed, as in Italy and Southern France, the hospitals were a great field for practical work, but we know little of the use made of them for clinical teaching. Of the English hospitals we must only mention two or three here.

St. Bartholomew's may be regarded as an instance of a great public city hospital for the cure of the sick attached to, but outside, a monastic house. Under Henry I., who gave the site in the year 1123, Rahere founded a Priory of Augustin Canons at Smithfield, and in their grounds a hospital dedicated to St. Bartholomew. Under the oversight of the Canons it was managed by a Master or Warden, eight brothers, and four sisters, and, after the pattern of the time, consisted of a large hall with cubicles for the sick, and small wards, chapels, and offices around it. Outside the hospital grounds there stretched a green moor, where races, jousts, and other sports took place. The hospital became quickly beloved by the citizens, and received a stream of benefactions ranging from lands and market tolls given by kings and nobles to the daily gifts of the butchers and artisans. To it flocked, say the chroniclers, sick and wounded men grieved with various diseases, sores, bleared eyes, epilepsy, dropsy, and palsies. For it was not an almshouse, but designed for the sick poor until such time as they recovered from their illness, and even for pregnant women during and after their confinements.

St. Thomas's Hospital was founded before 1207, when it was burnt down, rebuilt about 1213, again built on a fresh site in 1228. Later on it contained forty beds, and was managed by a Master and brethren and three lay sisters. The dedication

to St. Thomas à Becket was changed to St. Thomas
the Apostle, and after the dissolution it was once
more opened and re-endowed by the citizens and
King Edward VI. Under Charles II. it was used
for a time as a military hospital, and rebuilt about
1698 by Sir Robert Clayton and others.

St. Mary of Bethlehem, one of the first specialist
hospitals, was devoted to the care of the insane.
Its history is curious. In 1247 Simon FitzMary
founded a priory in Bishopsgate for the Bethlehem-
ite order, a body which consisted of hospitallers
attached to the great basilica at Bethlehem, and
possessing estates in France and Britain. It was
taken under the protection of the City in 1346, but
sequestrated as an alien priory two or three times
over, and apparently converted into a hospital for
lunatics about 1377. Dr. John Arundel, the
physician of Henry VI., and Dr. Thomas Deynman,
the physician of Henry VII., were two of its
Masters, and a gild of London citizens collected
a large part of its funds. In 1547 the hospital,
with the poor lunatics therein, was placed under
the control of the Corporation of London by
purchase from the Crown.

Miss Clay has collected some few facts about
other hospitals, such as St. Leonard's in York,
where 224 inmates were being cared for in 1370 ;
St. John at Canterbury, with one hundred beds; and

St. Bartholomew's at Gloucester, with forty beds. At York there was a matron and nurses, and one sister was described as Ann *Medica*. The Warden of such a hospital was, in some cases, a medical man, as at Preston in 1265, where Dr. Pascal de Bonona was Master; at Pontefract, where Dr. Louis Recouchez, a physician, was Warden. He later on was transferred to Westminster. In 1265 Magister Johannes, physicus, was acting as Master at Bridport. Another hospital of some standing was to be found at Lincoln, another possibly at Bristol, known as St. Mark's. The buildings of these institutions were usually in the form of a great hall, with rows of beds along the walls, and a chapel either at one end or detached. There were also small wards, and accommodation for the staff. Sometimes the buildings took the form of a quadrangle, or of two rows of houses with a narrow court between them, as we see in the Coventry almshouse.

Lazar Houses.—The leprosy epidemic in Europe was at its height from 1100 to 1350. Everywhere institutions sprang up for isolating and housing the lepers. Baas reckons some 1,900, and of these there were about 240 in England. As the outbreak died away the hospitals became useless, and many of them were converted to other purposes, such as schools and almshouses, by 1400. Queen Maud of Scotland and Bishop Hugh of Lincoln set a fashion of personally nursing and attending upon some of these unfortunates, who were carefully excluded from the towns and isolated by law. Thus there was a special form of writ, *De leproso amovendo*, and the leper lost the right to inherit property. Hence we find, besides Gilbert, John of Gaddesden about 1310, and Guy de Chauliac, 1363, discussing the importance of a true diagnosis. Some cures were attributed to the mineral waters at Bath and elsewhere. Indeed, there was a house at Bath for them founded by Saxon kings. John de Villula, a genial physician under William Rufus, the first Bishop of Bath, besides building a huge minster there, repaired the mineral springs and made two public baths ; while Bishop Reginald, of sporting proclivities, under Henry II., built the Hospital of St. John for the sick who flocked to the baths.

The Order of St. John of Jerusalem or the Knights Hospitallers deserves special mention. Some citizens of Amalfi founded a hospital at Jerusalem about 1013, and the order was constituted in 1113 *pro utilitate hominum*. Its work was twofold. It nursed the sick, and became in war the greatest bulwark of Christendom against the Saracens. Their splendid buildings in Jerusalem were taken over by Saladin in 1188, but their even grander hospital in Malta remains to-day, though

plundered of its contents by Napoleon. They were
established in Clerkenwell in 1101, and the first
buildings there date from 1185. All over England
their national branch or Langue formed com-
manderies, where their novices were trained, the
sick poor nursed, and the rents of their great estates
were collected. The Priory of Buckland Brewer in
Somerset was devoted to the use of the ladies and
serving sisters of the order in 1180, possibly the first
training school for nurses in England. To this Kil-
burn was afterwards added. Like other orders, the
English Langue was suppressed by Henry VIII.,
but it was revived in the nineteenth century under
royal patronage, and is the parent of the St. John
Ambulance Corps of to-day.

7. ANATOMY

Anatomy, which even in ancient times had been
a feeble plant, disappeared altogether after the
break-up of the Roman Empire. The Arabists
detested and abstained from it, and popular feeling
in Europe was equally against it, but in the school
of Salerno it began to revive (800-1200). At first
it was confined to the dissection of animals, and
Copho of Salerno wrote a popular handbook on the
anatomy of the pig. In the thirteenth century
lectures on anatomy by the great surgeons,
illustrated by diagrams and models, became

common. The leading authorities then were
Richard of Wendover, Canon of Westminster, an
English writer about 1252, and the surgeons
William Salicet and Henri de Mondeville. The
latter added a treatise on anatomy, with illustrations and diagrams, to his great work on surgery.
Actual dissection of the human body was carried
out by these surgeons and others. The study was
made compulsory for all students under the decree
of Frederick II., 1224, and soon after taken up in
the new universities.

8. The Organization of Surgeons

Besides the development of surgical and medical
study in the southern universities, we find that elsewhere in Europe the training and education of
surgeons was beginning to be regulated. We have
seen that in Salerno a seven years' course of study
was demanded, and that anatomy, practical work,
and examinations were the rule; but all Italy and,
later on, Spain and Germany came under an
Imperial decree in 1224 by which candidates for
medicine had to pass a public examination in Hippocrates, Galen, and Avicenna, must have studied
"logica" for three years, medicine and surgery for
five, and practised under an expert for a year. The
surgeon had to show that for at least a year he had

studied surgery, and in particular human anatomy, "without which no incision can safely be made, nor any fracture treated."

In France early in the same century the College of St. Côme arose, and aimed at creating a body of first-rate surgeons. In 1254 their Board of Examiners laid down that students must know Latin, spend two years at the university on medicine and philosophy, and two years in the study of surgery. Under the brilliant leading of Pitard, Lanfranc, and Mondeville an able body of surgeons grew up. We are not now concerned with the dreary history of their quarrels with the physicians, which lasted 450 years. Besides the graduates of St. Côme, there were numerous barber surgeons limited to minor operations only, and united into nineteen societies in the different towns. In England no records of surgical examination or organization have survived, but the barber surgeons now first appear, and later on became a curious legal corporation or corporations embracing every class and rank of surgeon, and sometimes physicians and apothecaries, forming a great public health service and the chief licensing bodies for the towns in surgery. This strange legal union of pure surgeons and barbers was confined to England, but "barber surgeons" existed elsewhere. What was their origin ? Both in ancient and modern times minor surgery had often been carried on by barbers. In Russia such men get a sort of licence to render first aid at the present day, and in Egypt Lord Kitchener had to issue regulations to improve the work of these old-established practitioners. In Germany the barber surgeons appeared as early as 1150, and were much in evidence. Under army customs there, down to recent times, the lower class of military surgeons, were called Feldscherers, and had to dress the hair and beards of the officers at least.

The numerous barber surgeons of the twelfth century in Western Europe were greatly increased by the endless bathing-houses which sprang up during the leprosy epidemic. The bath-keepers undertook shaving, bleeding, minor surgery, and massage for their customers, much in the same way as the Turkish baths to-day offer us massage, electrical, and manicure treatment. Then, too, the fashion of the time, leading physicians to disdain surgery, threw a good deal of practice into the hands of the barber surgeons, especially as the supply of military and other trained surgeons was small. However, they would have had little to do with the development of English surgery except for three causes : (1) They were numerous here just at the time of a socialistic revolution, the rise of the craft gilds, which converted the insignificant

individual barbers in a town into powerful gilds.
(2) The town authorities saw in these barbers'
gilds the means of forming a sort of sanitary
service in detecting plague and leprosy, and in
attending the wounded, and gave them power and
authority. Moreover, as Professor Ashley has
pointed out, such responsible gilds were a
guarantee of good work and a steady supply
of skilled craftsmen, who provided insurance for
themselves, education for their successors, and some
help for the sick poor. (3) All this might have
left them in their lowly condition, but for the
custom of linking up into one responsible gild all
sorts of different crafts. The pure surgeons,
amongst others, were thus linked up with barber
surgeons' gilds, and brought to them great functions
under the State. The central government created
them the licensing and educational authorities.
Further legal powers were given to the combined
body, so that for four centuries the history of
surgery in England is interwoven with that of these
gilds. In Florence thirty-six different trades, such
as mercers, artists, bookbinders, were sheltered
within the great medical gild, of which Dante, the
poet, was a member. The primary members of it
were physicians, surgeons, and apothecaries, but
the artists and mercers of the society shared in its
name and political privileges.

An extreme instance of the same thing exists here to-day in the City livery companies, where perhaps no one member exercises the craft which gives its name to a company, but in mediæval England the process went on even when the gilds were actively regulating the work of their members. About 1363 every man by law had to join a gild, and if his own craft had not one in the place, room must be found for him in another. Not only did various barber surgeon gilds include silk-weavers, cap-makers, chandlers, waferers, and rope-makers ; but also physicians, pure surgeons, and apothecaries are all to be found joined with them in course of tir. e in some places. In particular, the London gild from early times contained surgeons who practised nothing else, and after its union with the gild of military surgeons the legal powers granted to it did not apply to the non-surgical members, the barbers and others. Thus the barber surgeons' companies became a legal name or phrase for certain corporations in England to which most surgeons in practice had to belong down to the eighteenth century, while in France these companies contained no pure surgeons at all.

After the twelfth century, then, in England there were many barber surgeons beginning to form themselves into gilds and teaching their art to their apprentices.

3

NOTE ON THE GILD SYSTEM.—It may not be out of place here to consider these gilds which were so bound up with the organization of English surgery, and belong to a socialistic system of life differing entirely from the individualism of the last two centuries. It is difficult to realize the gulf which separates us from them. The elected authorities of the gild regulated every act of its members, and the gild had the monopoly of the trade or art in the place. It has taken three revolutions to destroy this social system. The abolition of the religious fraternities in the sixteenth century wiped out the voluntary communities in every place in which men exercised their religious life. Secondly, the paralysis in the early eighteenth century of the close trading corporations in every town set men free from their gilds to struggle as individual traders and capitalists without the old regulations. Thirdly, the old communal peasants, with their common field system, were finally extinguished under the Enclosure Acts.

The craft gilds were one part of this system, and became common in the middle of the thirteenth century. The weavers in London and a few others formed their little societies at the beginning of the century. The date of the first barbers' gild is unknown, but when the Inquisition of 1387 compelled a return of the existing gilds and their property, the reply was made for some barbers' gilds that they had existed "from a time to which the memory of man goeth not." This afterwards became a legal phrase for the reign of Richard I., but it is doubtful whether that meaning attached to it then, and there is strong evidence against gilds of a single craft being common in the period 1189-1199.

Religious and social gilds arose in far earlier times in such numbers that we find 909 in Norfolk alone, but these included men of various occupations. Again, the single *merchant gilds* in a town under the Plantagenet kings often formed the first bond of union, and were merged into or replaced by the new city corporations. Gross has traced them in 162 towns, where they protected the trading rights of the burghers from outsiders and from the semi-free populace. They aimed at a monopoly of the trade of the place, and at protection of the burghers when travelling elsewhere. Under their shelter, men of each separate trade about 1250 began to form the *craft gilds* for members of their own trade. The fashion spread everywhere, and even in tiny towns the few practitioners of each art were expected to form their own gild or join with another. Thus, in Hull, the Merchant Venturers, the Gild of St. George, the Merchants of the Staple, and perhaps the Weavers' and Gold-smiths' Gilds, appear about 1300. The Barbers'

Gild in London is found in 1308 under a warden, though it may have existed fifty years earlier.   Such a society, modelled on the old social gilds, combined religious and social functions with the regulation of its craft, and under the protection of the merchant gild or corporation shared indirectly in the government of the town.   Just as at the present day "the recognition of a Trades Union" is often a burning question, so in the first half of the fourteenth century it was all-important for a gild to get recognized as holding the monopoly of the trade and the right of regulating the work and behaviour of its members.   The chief gilds did get this monopoly, but with certain reservations, lest they should interfere with the food and other necessities of life for the community.   Thus, besides the supervision of their rules by the town authorities, "open fair days" and markets were ordained, when "foreigners"—*i.e.*, men living outside—could come in and compete freely with the city craftsmen. The country surgeon or the travelling clothier or armourer could for some hours practise their avocation in the town, while for the rest of the week they were liable to penalties if they treated or dealt with the citizens.   Hence the importance of obtaining the freedom of the city, which was a licence to practise or trade in it, and granted only to members of a gild or company.

CHAPTER II

1300 TO 1500 A.D.

1. THE POSITION OF SURGERY IN EUROPE AND AT HOME

THE advance of the art was slower than in the earlier period. At first the great schools of surgery in Italy fell off for a time, but Montpellier and Paris grew and flourished exceedingly. The teaching of Guy de Chauliac, Mondeville, Pitard, and their successors shows the high standard reached. Then the Universities of Bologna, Padua, and Florence came to the front, and became centres of teaching and research which towards the later half of the fifteenth century was greatly increased by the revival of classical studies and the influx of Greek refugee teachers and their libraries. Even before this revival Peter of Argelata and Bertapaglia had made great reputations.

Guy de Chauliac, a poor peasant boy from the Auverne, became the greatest authority on surgery in Europe. He had studied at Toulouse, Montpellier, and Paris, worked at anatomy in Bologna, became canon and prior of the church of St. Justus, and an honoured attendant of three popes. At Avignon he saw and suffered from the Black Death—the bubonic plague—while other men ran away. His chief work, *The Great Surgery*, appeared soon after 1363, and was the favourite textbook for a long period. While it shows his wide knowledge of Greek and Arabist authors, he is not afraid of criticizing them and of recommending recent improvements, whether by himself or by others. Speaking of ancient writers, he says " we are like children sitting on the neck of a giant who see all that he sees and something besides " (Withington, *Medical History*, p. 217). Unfortunately this Prince of Surgeons, as Freind calls him, opposed the Listerianism of Theodoric, and hindered its adoption; but he is excellent on fractures of the skull, and, indeed, on fractures and dislocations generally. He incised and drained empyemata and recommended the long splint with a pulley and weight for extension in fractured femur. Curiously enough, the existing fashion in English hospitals of a rope or chain hanging over the patient's bed by which he can raise or turn himself easily, as well as the bandages stiffened by white of egg, are due to his inventive mind and care for details. His treatise, says Allbutt, " is rich, aphoristic, orderly, and precise." The radical cure of hernia was one of

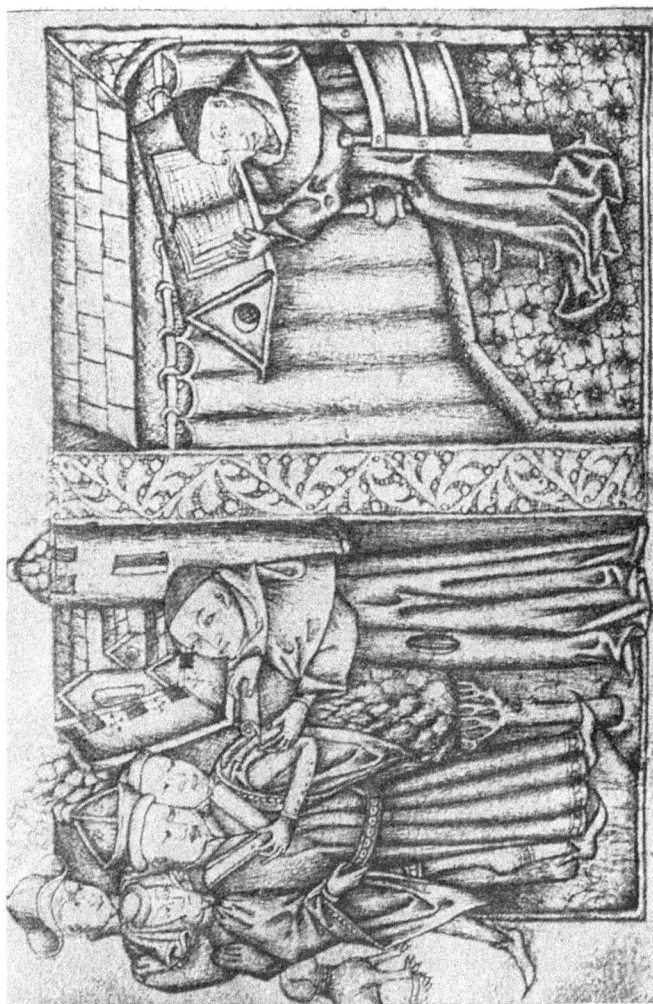

FRONTISPIECE OF THE UNIQUE BRISTOL COPY OF GUY DE CHAULIAC'S "SURGERY."

Made by John Tourtier at the request of the Duke of Bedford when Regent of France, with an English Glossary, etc., for the use of English Surgeons, about 1422.

the operations which he rescued from the quacks
of the time, and to him we owe the account of the
narcotic inhalation used as an anæsthetic for a
long period.

Peter of Argelata (died 1423), a professor at
Bologna, was another brilliant surgeon, but preferred drying powders to the spirit lotions of
Theodoric. He employed drainage-tubes of per-
forated metal, and trephined both the skull and long
bones. To *Bertapaglia*, a professor at Padua, we
owe the plan of drawing out and isolating a vessel
before ligaturing it, and the suture of the intestines
by catgut and the glover's stitch. At Padua, too,
began the fashion of issuing " *consilia*," which were
published discussions on selected cases or consultations by eminent teachers. Many of these had a
wide circulation, like the aphorisms and letters of
Boerhaave in later days. Montagnana of Padua
was the first of these writers, and one of the earliest
to read the original Greek texts when brought to
Italy.

The times, however, were less propitious than
the preceding age. The Black Death in 1349 had
swept away half the population of Europe ; the
schism of the papacy and political unrest, and the
gradual advance of the Saracen host, submerging
and destroying year by year more and more of the
eastern states of Europe, seem to have sapped the

energy of the western races. It was the same in Britain. All the activity in literary, artistic, and political thought vanished with the Black Death; and the rest of the period was filled with the Hundred Years' War, the struggle between different classes, different religions, and different claimants for the throne. The wars, however, compelled some attention to military surgery, and continental intercourse and influence was undiminished. At the beginning of the period Edward I. ruled over an empire extending from Aberdeen to Bordeaux, and both then and later English students went to and fro constantly to the Italian and French schools.

Greater care of the soldiers in the field became apparent from the formation of army medical corps and ambulances. Indeed, the military surgeons became a distinct class in Europe. Charles the Bold, Duke of Burgundy, seems to have appointed a surgeon to each company in his army, and this number of surgeons continued to be the recognized rule till about 1655, when the custom began of attaching one surgeon to each regiment.

The ambulances created by the humanity of Isabella of Castile about 1470 were the forerunners of a movement which has been enormously extended in our own time. She provided six large tents with furniture, physicians, surgeons, orderlies, and medicines not only for the wounded, but for all soldiers suffering from disease. At the siege of Granadas she got together 400 covered waggons or *ambulancias* to carry out the removal of the wounded, and, what is more remarkable, she organized a large body of skilled nurses of good character under strict supervision to attend to them. The good results as to the health of the armies and the encouragement of the soldiers, who saw themselves well looked after if ill or wounded, became apparent to all, and led, though by slow steps (Mostyn Bird, *The Errand of Mercy;* Pedro Boscar, and others), to the subsequent development of the system.

2. The Chief English Surgeons

Though we produced no men of the first rank such as Chauliac and Theodoric, a number of able operators and skilled surgeons are found. Of Morstead we shall speak later; Ferris, though renowned as a teacher, left no writings behind him ; but some fuller account must be given of Arderne and Mirfield.

John of Arderne is one of the very few English surgeons of the time who wrote on professional matters, and he is one of whom any country may be proud. Sir D'Arcy Power rightly says that he was a scholar and a gentleman, a man of good education, wide experience, and sound judgment.

If he shows sometimes a liking for astrology and charms, it does not affect his care in studying the right way to do an operation. It was a concession to the fashion of the day.

He was born in 1307, and seems to have served under two Dukes of Lancaster in succession—at Antwerp, at Algeciras in Spain, and also in Aquitaine. For twenty years he practised at Newark, and came to London in 1370, where he joined the Gild of Military Surgeons, with a high reputation among the princely and noble families of that brilliant era of chivalry, knowing personally, as he did, "so many of the peerless knights and splendid champions who survive in the pages of Froissart." Some of them he mentions by name as his patients, and others he refers to by their coats of arms. He is the only contemporary authority for the story how the Prince of Wales obtained the ostrich feather, "which that most noble Lord King [of Bohemia] had used hitherto to bear above his crest." He employed the leisure of his latter days to publish treatises such as *The Care of the Eyes*, on *Venesection*, on *Sinuses and Fistulæ in Ano*, on *The Use of Rectal Injections*, on *Plants and their Uses*, and a commentary on Giles de Corbeil's book on the urine, as well as a *Scala Sanitatis contra Plagas*. These were widely read textbooks for many years. In the treatise on

Afterward I cured sir Reynald Grey.
lord of Ruthyn in Walez and lord of
Schirlond byside Chestfeld whiche
asked consel at þe moste famose lechez
of Ingland and none availed hym
Afterward I cured sir Henry Blakborne
clerk Tresorere of þe lord Prince of
Walez. Afterward I cured Adam Omwfr
of Schelford byside Nottinghm and
sir John preste of þe same toune
and John of Holle of Schirlande
and sir Thos Hamelden psone of
Langar in þe vale of Benare.
Afterward I heled sir John ayasty
psone of Stafforto i chestre shire
Afterward I cured frere Thos Gunn
custode of þe frere aynos of Zork
Afterward in þe zere of o lord 1340.
I come to london and þ Iames John
Colyn ayare of Northampton þ asked
consel at many lechez Afterward
I heled or cured Wel deinn ffysk
maugur of london in Bugge strete

)

Sinuses he says : " In that year when our strenuous and warlike Prince [of Wales] departed unto God, I wrote this little book of mine with my own hand "—viz., in the year 1376.   As an operator his fees were high ; he says that he had never done his operation for fistula for less than £100 in our money, but, he adds, let another man do as he thinks best and most suitable.   He is delightful when he chats as a botanist about the places where juniper grows in Kent and in Surrey, where the people call it gorst because they do not know its proper name ; or, again, where he gives the names he had picked up in different countries for sundry common plants.

He devised a carefully thought out operation for fistula in ano, which was a modification of that of Albucasis.   He placed his patient in the lithotomy position.   Then he first passed a probe threaded with a fourfold ligature through the fistula into the rectum, and drew out one end of the ligature through the anus and tied the two ends together. A grooved director was next passed through the fistula and a shield introduced into the rectum. After drawing the ligature tight, a scalpel was passed along the director, and with a single movement the director, scalpel, and shield were drawn out to-gether, dividing the fistula from end to end.   The bleeding was stopped by sponges wrung out in warm water, and by making the patient sit on the sponge as a pad. Afterwards he dressed the wound with dry, clean pads and a powder, held in place by a **T** bandage. All irritative dressings were avoided and enemata of oil given daily.

It is worth noticing how he reiterates his warnings not to mistake a cancer of the rectum for a simple ulceration. "Explore carefully with the finger at any rate, and," he adds, "do not be led away and offer to operate. It will only be a disgrace to you. Warn the friends of the certain ending."

The following is a brief abstract of his chapter on cancer of the rectum. A bubo is a tumour developing in the rectum, of great hardness, but with little pain at first. It is nothing but a hidden cancer, and is called bubo from an owl, because that bird lurks in darkness. It is diagnosed by the surgeon putting his finger into the rectum where he finds a mass of stony hardness, sometimes on one side, sometimes on both, which hinders the passage of fæces. After a time it ulcerates out, and may even destroy the sphincter. The patient is driven to stool two or three times an hour to relieve the aching and darting pain. The stools are ill-smelling and streaked with watery blood. Ignorant doctors and patients think it is a dysentery, which it certainly is not. A dysentery is a diarrhœa, but cancer produces hard stools, which sometimes cannot pass the obstruction and may require

removal by the finger.   Ignorant people give medicines, which increase the constipation and harden
the scybala.   He used simple enemata of bran water
or mallows, without oil, fat, or butter, because fatty
substances feed the cancer.

The patients at first go about as usual.   They eat
very little and have frequent urgent calls to stool.
They often die towards autumn, and, when failing,
they show a slight fever and lose appetite more
and more every day, only craving for ale or wine.
They sleep uneasily and are heavy in mind and
body.   Finally, growing very feeble, they remain in
bed and take little but water.   Then death is at
the gates.

The simple injections alleviate greatly the dis-
comfort, but beware above all things that you do not
undertake to operate, and warn the friends or the
patient that it is incurable.

The finger in the rectum if dysentery is present
feels nothing but what is found in the healthy, but
if a cancer exists there is a swelling, very hard, of
the size of a hen's egg or larger.   The discharge in
both diseases, during defæcation or apart from it,
is much the same.   In dysentery there is pain
about the navel or in the flanks.   In cancer this is
absent, but there is darting or aching pain and
tenesmus.   He concludes:

" I have never seen nor heard of any man who

recovered from cancer, but I have known many who died of it."

His instructions to surgeons show a higher moral tone than that of some of his predecessors. He exhorts his brethren to cultivate modesty, charity, and particularly a studious, chaste habit of life in word and deed. Thus he tells them that—

He that would succeed in this art should always set God before him in all his doings, and with heart and soul call for His help. He should not be rash or boastful in his words or deeds, and should refrain from much talk, especially among men of rank, but answer questions warily lest he be entrapped in his words. In fact, if his deeds are often found to differ from his words, he will be held of little worth and will blemish his good reputation.

He must not be too much given to laughter or sport, and, as much as he can, he should flee the company of knaves and dishonest people, and always be occupied in things relating to his art. He should either write, or study, or pray, for the study of books is an honour to a leech. Above everything, he must be always sober, for drunkeness destroys all virtue and brings it to nought. Let him learn to be content in strange places with the meat and drink to be found there, using measure in everything. He should scorn no one. If another doctor is spoken of, he should neither decry him nor praise him unduly, but he may courteously answer, " I have not much knowledge of him, but I have neither learned nor heard anything of him but what was good and honourable."

He must be chaste in word and deed, and he should be guarded in handling and gazing on the wives and daughters or other fair women in great men's houses, lest he cause anger in their relatives. He should avoid giving annoyance to servants. To patients who come to him he should neither be too familiar nor too ungracious. He should not be too ready to undertake every case which offers, and always see it before doing so, and fix his fees, which should not be unduly low. Patients should not be led to expect a cure before a reasonable time. If they do get well very early, you can tell them that it is their good constitution, for they are very delighted to hear that. The surgeon should take care to be well dressed, not like a minstrel, but in habit and bearing like a " clerke," for a prudent man in clerkly attire may sit at any gentleman's table. He must have clean hands, well-shapen nails, neither black nor dirty, and, when at a great man's table, he must be courteous and take care that no act or word of his annoy the guests. He should hear much and speak little. When he does speak, it should be

as well expressed and reasonable as he can, avoiding
all bad language and want of candour. Let him
learn, too, how to comfort his patients with wise
reflections, and, indeed, with merry tales. He
must never disclose the confidences of his patients,
whether men or women, nor, indeed, speak ill of
anyone, even if he has reason to do so. If a patient
sees that he keeps other people's secrets, he will
naturally put more confidence in him.

John of Mirfield is another writer of this period
who should be remembered as a worthy represent-
ative of the university and hospital class. It is
probable that he had been a student of medicine
at Oxford under Tyngewich, the physician of
Edward I., but the details of his early life are
obscure. He was apprenticed to a master of
whom, according to Sir Norman Moore, he speaks
with much respect and veneration, and he attained
an honourable position as member of the staff of
St. Bartholomew's Hospital, and canon of the
Priory which governed it. This hospital was, even
then, an old and prominent institution for the cure
of the sick, and not merely an almshouse. Its
situation, close to the great tournament ground of
Smithfield, was convenient for the treatment of
the wounded. He was a contemporary of John
of Arderne, but his quiet and semi-monastic life
stands in strong contrast with Arderne's, and his

work did not bring him into such close contact
with royal and military celebrities. In 1380 he
wrote a treatise on medicine and surgery embody-
ing much of his experience in practice, the *Breviarium Bartolomei*, divided into fifteen sections.
The ninth section discusses wounds and bruises;
the tenth takes up fractures, dislocations, and twists
of bones; and the eleventh is occupied with dislocations of joints. He is not afraid to fix with
precision how long each fracture ought to take for
complete union. A rib, he finds, requires twenty
days, a humerus or femur forty; and he holds that
union is more difficult in the aged. Certain dislocations are to be reduced by an instrument *quod
vocatur tornellus*, in English wyndas. (*The Progress of Medicine at St. Bartholomew's Hospital*,
p. 18, Norman Moore.)

His chief reputation is based on his teaching
as a physician, and the occasional notes of cases
which he gives show observation and thought as
well as book knowledge. As a clerk and canon
he was, of course, in minor orders, but it is doubtful whether he entered the priesthood. In fact,
he was assessed for taxation as a layman, and it
is probable that his ecclesiastical status did not
prevent him practising surgery. Indeed, he protests
against the fashionable division of medicine and
surgery in these spirited words :

4

" Long ago, unless I mistake, physicians used to practise surgery, but nowadays there is a great distinction between surgery and medicine, and this, I fear, arises from pride, because physicians disdain to work with their hands, though, indeed, I myself have a suspicion that it is because they do not know how to perform particular operations ; and this unfortunate usage has led the public to believe that a man cannot know both subjects, but the well informed are aware that he cannot be a good physician who neglects every part of surgery, and, on the other hand, a surgeon is good for nothing who is without knowledge of medicine."

It is a great thing to find at this time a leader of medical thought protesting against this unfortunate division, which has done so much to hinder progress, to sterilize medicine, and to degrade surgery.

3. Organization of Surgery in England

The Military Surgeons may first be noticed. The demand for them in the Hundred Years' War and the struggle of the Roses must have been enormous. The conflict in France was not a savage, tribal fight, but English gold supported large bodies of well-paid troops whose lives and health had a money value. Under the system of ransoms, even prisoners were worth the utmost care and attention, and thus surgeons were almost as important as artillery, equipments, and transport.

An oft-quoted document of 1415 shows Henry V. agreeing with his physician, Nicolas Colnet, and his surgeon, Thomas Morstead, to undertake the care of his army in the expedition of Agincourt. Morstead's pay was, with a hundred marks a quarter and a share of booty, to be about sixteen shillings a day in our money, and he was to have as lieutenant William Bredwardine and twelve surgeons, who got the equivalent of eight shillings a day each, together with their share of the plunder. These surgeons were accordingly impressed for service.

Sir D'Arcy Power has shown that the higher ranks of these surgeons were united in a small society in London of fifteen to twenty members, who in 1369, if not earlier, obtained some recognition from the city and existed for two centuries. Of their temporary alliance with the physicians and struggles with the barber surgeons, and the final amalgamation of the two bodies, we shall speak later on.

When the rules of this Gild of Military Surgeons were revised in 1435, they had only seventeen men, including the two old comrades, Morstead and Bredwardine. St. Luke's Day was fixed for their annual dinner and church parade, but the general business meeting was earlier in the year, on the feast of St. Cosmo and St. Damian, the great patron saints of the medical art. As the

barber surgeon society had four Masters, two
for each craft, the Military Gild determined to
have four also, a really liberal allowance for the
seventeen; but the office was no sinecure, for it
was laid down that a consultation with a Master
must be held over every major operation. Apprentices were to serve six years and then pass an examination. If they failed, they could do another
six years and try again, but failure then disqualified
them for ever from entering the sacred circle. The
plan had at least the merit of simplicity. If a
surgeon took an assistant, the gild examined his
knowledge within a month, and if he passed he
could enter on a three years' agreement. Was an
assistantship the fate of the "chronic" student, or
were they qualified men who had not the freedom
of the city or capital sufficient to start for themselves? Finally, it was laid down that the great
seventeen should always give each other assistance,
and should not filch each other's patients.

With exception of John of Arderne, none of
these highly placed surgeons seem to have made
any name for themselves in literature. After
Morstead's death John Ferris appears to have had
the greatest professional reputation, and was long
revered. The Civil Wars dragged their weary
course along, and afforded an ample field for the
surgeon. In the later years of the period the best

students went to Italy to listen to the lectures of
the Humanists, bringing back a scientific spirit
for research as well as an enthusiasm for classical
literature. Among the lecturers in Italy we may
recall the name of John Free of Balliol, who
lectured at Florence, Padua, and Ferrara, and translated one or more of the classical medical writers.

The Act of 1421.—It must be remembered that
the barber surgeon companies' jurisdiction was, as
a rule, limited to the towns, and though surgeons
taught by them or by the universities or monasteries or in foreign schools were found practising
in country districts, still there was no means of
putting down ignorant pretenders of all kinds.
Parliament took up the matter in 1421, after the
Treaty of Troyes had apparently ended the French
wars.

As Dr. J. A. Nixon has pointed out, this was
*the first law regulating the practice of medicine and
surgery in England.* A petition was presented
to Parliament praying that no one should be allowed
to practise physic unless he had studied in the
school of physic in some university, and graduated
in the same as Bachelor or Doctor of Medicine,
under pain of imprisonment and a fine of £40 to
the King ; that no woman should practise physic ;
that the sheriff of every shire should search for
offenders in his circuits; and, lest anyone who is

really qualified should be excluded, that every practitioner who has not graduated should appear on a
fixed date and be admitted to a degree if he passes
a thorough examination in some university.   The
Parliament, instead of a statute, enacted that the
King's Council should have authority to legislate
by ordinance (see Stubbs, *Constitutional History*,
ii. 584) against unqualified practitioners of medicine
and of surgery.   The Norman-French text may be
thus translated (*Rotuli Parliam.*, vol. iv., pp. 130,
158, ix., Henry V.): Item on account of various
mischiefs and dangers which have existed a long
while among the people of this kingdom, because
some of those who use the arts and practice of
medicine and surgery pretend that they are well
and sufficiently learned in the said arts, whereas in
truth they have no standing, to the great deception
of the people :—Be it both ordained and agreed to
by this Parliament that the Lords of the King's
Council for the time being shall have power and
authority from the same Parliament to make and
put forth suitable ordinances and penalties against
those persons in future who shall occupy and use
the practice of the aforesaid arts, and yet are neither
skilled nor approved as qualified in the same arts—
that is to say, the practitioners of physic by the
universities, and the surgeons by the masters of
that art ; and this shall be done as shall seem

suitable and necessary to the said Lords according to their discretion and judgment. (Robert Hare renders it : " Ne quis exerceat practicam in artibus medicinæ et chirurgiæ nisi prius in universitatibus fuerit approbatus—viz., in medicina apud universitates et in chirurgia apud magistros ejusdem artis.") The phrase "les mestres de cett Arte" would include both the university officials and those of the legal gilds.   We know nothing of the measure of success which followed, but a hundred years later fresh legislation against the plague of quacks was necessary.   For the meantime the education and organization of surgeons was left by the State to local bodies.

The Barber Surgeons.—It has been shown that the British barber surgeon gilds became important about 1800, retaining many features of the old religious and social gilds, but gaining power from the system of craft gilds with their monopolies, and still more as time went on from their inclusion of pure surgeons.   They thus became the chief licensing bodies for the towns, and exercised a strict control over their members' practice.   In the best of these gilds the purely surgical section built up an excellent system of education partly by the old apprenticeship and partly by lectures, examinations and anatomical teaching.   It was chiefly in this period that they became the legal corporations, which included, educated, and licensed nearly the whole of British surgeons for 400 years. Most of their records have perished, but they can be traced in more than twenty-five towns, and their ordinances in about twelve different places still exist, showing great variety of structure from the simple barber craft gild up to the great surgical corporations in London and three or four other towns, each with a separate and somewhat oppressed section of barbers, waferers, and others linked to them. It is clear that their members were many, for the London society at one time (1527) outnumbered every other city company. Only one barber surgeon company still has a legal existence—that of Newcastle—where ten members have the freedom by inheritance, and are ruled by two stewards, pointing to their former division into surgeons and barbers. Of course, under the present Act of 1858 they have no licensing powers, even if they had kept up their old lectures and examinations.

We have seen, too, that the Act of 1363 compelled every surgeon to belong to one of these gilds, and another of 1387 enforced a return of their rules and property, while a third fixed apprenticeship at seven years. They had not only a monopoly of practice, but the power of regulating the work of their members by insisting on consultations in

important cases and general efficiency. A further
step in State regulation took place in 1436, when
a statute enacted that the ordinances of surgical
and all other gilds must be submitted for the
approbation of the magistrates of each city, and
accordingly we find this municipal licensing of the
surgeon and barber gilds, in London, York, Bristol,
Newcastle, Salisbury, Exeter, and Durham. Indeed, the date of this approbation is often taken to
be that of the foundation of the gild, which had
existed long before. After the inspection and
ratification the rules were enforced by the city
authorities by fine or imprisonment.

A final step is seen in the Charters and special
Acts of Parliament which in later times completed
the State Regulation, though the licensing bodies
remained numerous. Thus the London company
got a Royal Charter in 1462, Henry VI. gave one
to Dublin in 1446 to " establish the art of surgery,"
and Edinburgh obtained one in 1506.

The London gild was " recognized " by the city
in 1308, and their Master, Richard, was sworn to
supervise their practice. Two years later one of
them, Gerard, possibly the Master, was placed in
charge of Newgate to examine new-comers so as to
prevent lepers entering the city. We quickly find
evidence that they were becoming divided into
surgeons on the one hand, and barbers and others

in a second group; as Sir James Paget remarks, "there always were surgeons distinct from the barbers from first to last, even during their temporary conjunction "[by law]. From 1376 they were ruled by four Masters, or two Masters and two wardens, in consequence of the dual character of the gild. In the returns of 1388 their ordinances tell us nothing of their work, but mention their ethical committee for deciding disputes; their pensions to decayed members of £2. 5s. 6d. per annum, perhaps £30 in our money; and their rule against taking away each other's assistants. Lectures in surgery began to be given about 1350, and in the next century definite provision for education, not only by apprenticeship, but by special teachers, examiners in surgery, and then masters, readers, and demonstrators of anatomy are found who included the best men of the day. The first diploma now extant is one granted to Robert Anson after a public examination on August 1, 1497, by Master John Smith, Doctor in Physic, instructor and examiner of the Fellowship of Barbers and Surgeon Barbers, in the presence of many experts. It recites that their charter had given them the right of examination, and disciplinary powers over freemen of the city and over foreigners—*i.e.*, persons from outside—practising any part of surgery in London, and that the said Robert Anson had now been examined in the operative and directive (practical and theoretical) parts of the science and art of surgery, and found able and discreet. He is therefore licensed both as to the treatment of new wounds, cancers, fistulas, etc., and authorized to practise in every place. From a reference to his previous skill it seems possible that he was a new-comer, and not an apprentice in London. Mr. Young seems to think that women, too, were also allowed to qualify.

This gild fellowship or company fought fiercely with the gild of military surgeons for the right of supervision over everyone practising surgery. The city corporation inclined sometimes to one side, sometimes to the other, but the barber surgeons eventually won. Decisions in favour of the military men were given in 1369 and 1390, and in favour of their opponents in 1376, 1410, and 1415, when the city appointed the Masters, and punished all offenders against their rules, especially as to anyone who did not seek a consultation with one of the Masters for any patient in serious danger. The military surgeons next made an alliance with the London physicians to form an *Academy of Medicine* which would take away the licensing powers of the universities and of the barber surgeon gild in London. They accordingly presented a petition to the mayor and aldermen that the physicians and surgeons in the city might be formed into a society, governed by a Rector of Medicine, two surveyors of the faculty of physic, and two Masters of the craft of surgery. This was granted in May, 1423. They arranged for three houses to be thrown together to form their examination hall and lecture rooms. It was decided that their officers should be elected annually, the Rector being, if possible, a Doctor of Physic, Master of Arts and Philosophy, and as their first nominee they chose Gilbert Kymer, who was afterwards Chancellor of Oxford. All surgeons were to be examined and approved by the Rector, the two Masters, and the majority of the craft, and were then to be licensed by the mayor and alder-men. All major cases were to have the benefit of consultation with the Rector and one of the Masters without payment; malpraxis was to be punished by the mayor; the drugs of the apothecaries were to be inspected, and the poor treated gratuitously. It was an attractive scheme. Whether Mr. Morstead, the old army surgeon, had picked up the idea from Paris or elsewhere, he and Mr. J. Harvey were made Masters in surgery, and the great scheme was launched. But the barber surgeons took fright and appealed again to the corporation, showing that the academy was a denial of their privileges. The city replied that they had not intended to interfere with them, and that their powers were inviolable (1424).

There was clearly no room for the two authorities, and the academy quickly came to an end.

After this failure the military surgeons gave up the attempt to crush out their rivals, and the latter occupied themselves in developing their educational system. They succeeded in getting from Edward IV. their first charter in 1462, which contains much about surgery and hardly mentions the barbers. It granted them exemption from service on juries, and full powers over all "exercising" surgery, and the right to examine and approve them. They had previously obtained the corporation's approbation of their ordinances in 1451 according to the Act of 1436, and this was repeated after the charter in 1482 and 1487. As their powers were now so secure, the military surgeons came to an agreement with them in 1498 by *The Composition*, which laid down that two Wardens of each society should together examine and try all aliens, strangers, and foreigners, who shall not practise till allowed by the four Wardens. The members of each society shall not be allowed to change to the other, but the Wardens shall rule both and act as consultants. Mutual help shall be given by advice and co-operation.

Thus the union of all surgeons in London was carried out, to be finally completed by an Act of Parliament in 1540, a striking contrast to the state of things in Paris, where the quarrels between the

College of St. Côme and the barber surgeons continued till the eighteenth century.

The York Gild.—Dr. Auden mentions that the city of York in 1345 sent two barber surgeons, William of Bolton and Hugh of Kelvinton, all the way to Bamborough to treat a political prisoner, David Bruce, and to extract the arrow with which he had been wounded at the battle of Neville's Cross. These surgeons received a fee of about £90 in our money for their services. The earliest form of the gild ordinances dates from about 1400, but this was revised 1486: apprentices after seven years were examined and not permitted to practise till they had passed; strangers coming into the city were subject to similar tests, and prevented from practising if found inefficient.

The Oxford Gild was incorporated by the Chancellor of the University, Dr. Northwood, in 1348, and besides surgeons included barbers and waferers, to whom hurers were added in 1499 by Cardinal Morton under the condition that each body practised its own craft only. Under their rules surgeons were ordered to get consultations in all difficult cases, and never to reveal the diseases of their patients. No one might practise surgery or the other crafts of the gild except under the supervision and permission of their officials. No surgeon might take over another man's patient unless the

previous attendant "be contented to leave his
cure." If the Master was not a surgeon he should
not act as consultant. No one who was not duly
apprenticed might be taught surgery unless he gave
a bond not to practise within twenty miles.

There is little of surgical interest in the surviving
records of the gilds in Lincoln (founded 1369),
Newcastle, Durham, Exeter, Salisbury, Bristol
(existing 1395), Norwich, Chester, and other places
in this period, though several of them are found
soon after engaged in educational work. Dublin,
Aberdeen, and Edinburgh afford equally scanty
materials.

4. THE HOSPITALS

The great movement for building hospitals had
lasted two hundred years, and Europe was now
covered with institutions of the kind lavishly
endowed. The details of construction were improved, and some of the finest edifices of the day
were those designed for hospitals in the chief cities.
In the greater monasteries, too, elaborate arrangements for the supply of hot and cold water,
drainage, sanitary arrangements, and warm rooms
for the sick were provided, although the sanitary
condition of private houses and the streets of the
towns was neglected to the last degree. The
hospitals of the Holy Ghost in most cities under

municipal control were the pride of the citizens and gave relief to vast numbers. Garrison refers particularly to the technical care devoted to the construction of the great hospital at Milan, which was not completed till 1456, but everywhere similar institutions were erected with all the skill that the science of the time could provide. As the leprosy outbreak had come to an end in most places, some of the 1,900 leper houses were turned into general hospitals and others sold or used as almshouses for the poor. At the same time, too, the public bathing houses, which were almost as prominent in mediæval times as in Rome or Japan, began to go out of fashion, till in the sixteenth and seventeenth centuries they vanish altogether except at a few mineral spas.

5. The Universities

The Italians were still increasing the number of university schools, and the Princes of various cities patronized what had been a purely popular movement. Padua, Florence, and other cities rivalled the older universities and attracted students from all parts. Montpellier continued to be one of the greatest centres of surgical and medical teaching. The British universities, though their colleges and students were constantly increasing, certainly gained no renown in surgery. Clifford Allbutt thinks that they excluded it altogether, but, as a matter of fact, the records of the English universities are scanty, and it is quite possible that surgery was definitely taught.   Men like Mirfield seem to have studied surgery as well as medicine at the university, and towards the end of the period we find a definite course of surgical study mentioned and examinations held.

6. ANATOMY

The revival of the practice of human dissection in the thirteenth century, and the importance attributed to it by the great writers on surgery, led to the regular study of the subject everywhere during these two centuries, but no great advance in knowledge was made.   It has been said in explanation that the uncritical habit of accepting the teaching of classical writers as true led men to overlook or disbelieve the actual facts which presented themselves to the dissector.   At any rate, we do not find a single accurate anatomical drawing until the time of Leonardo da Vinci and the other contemporary artists.   These men, however, made it their business to represent exactly what they saw.   The result is perfectly true to nature, and does not give the bones and muscles which Galen said should be there.   Galen, by the way, seems to have chiefly dissected animals.   All this is strange if it be a true explanation of the slow progress of the art, yet every Italian surgeon, as we have seen, had to study anatomy from the year 1224, if not earlier. Mundinus at Bologna wrote a feeble but popular students' handbook in 1316, but it happens that no really able treatise on the subject in the whole period has survived, though Chauliac and other great surgeons speak so strongly about dissection. Buck states that Leonardo's drawings were made from the dissections of Della Torre of Verona, who died before he could publish his great work on anatomy. He mentions, too, Gabriel Zerbi as another able anatomist of the time. Berengario de Carpi, again, claims that he had dissected 100 bodies. Public dissections were regularly given in most universities, notably at Venice from 1308; Montpellier, 1366; Florence, 1388; Lerida, 1391; Vienna, 1404; Bologna, 1405; Padua, 1429; Prague, 1460; Paris, 1478; and Tübingen, 1485. An oft-mentioned Papal Bull of 1300 was not intended to hinder scientific dissections, but merely forbade a fashion of eviscerating and boiling the bodies of dead Crusaders in order to transport them to Europe. In England there is no record surviving of the formal institution of dissections at the universities, but they are spoken of as a matter of course when in the sixteenth century a list appears of the lectures and work required from candidates for a licence. Vicary's textbook in 1577 seems, according to Dr. Payne, to have really been a revised edition of an old fifteenth century anatomical students' handbook, possibly the usual one employed at the earliest barber surgeons' lectures.

Pathological anatomy was studied by at least one great writer, Benivieni of Florence (1448-1512), who has left interesting descriptions of biliary calculus, hip-joint disease, ruptured bowel, scirrhus of the pylorus, stenosis of the intestine, and other subjects (Clifford Allbutt, *Historical Relations*, p. 58).

CHAPTER III

1500 TO 1600 A.D.

1. GENERAL SURVEY OF THE TIME

IT is natural to expect great changes in the sixteenth century, for the Renaissance, the Reformation, the printing press, the discovery of America,
and the Tudor autocracy led to a revolution in the
whole of social life. Natural science as well as
classical literature now became an object of
enthusiastic study. In the last chapter we saw
how Englishmen, like Free, Linacre, Caius and
Grocyn travelled to Italy to study the Greek writers;
and the movement continued. This in itself was
enough to start a revival in medicine and surgery,
but there was more to come. The scientific spirit
for research and for testing evidence was developed,
and new exact sciences sprang to life under this
mental awakening. Men were no longer content
to learn what Galen and Avicenna had said on
anatomy and physiology. By patient experiment
and dissections they sought out what the facts
actually were and founded practically new sciences.

It was soon felt that students must themselves practise actual dissections if their surgery was not to be merely haphazard, and, accordingly, dissections became part of their ordinary training.   Chemistry, mechanics, and mathematics became also objects of study, and the results were soon found applicable to medicine, surgery, and physiology.   The discovery of the strange plants and animals of America had its effect in starting afresh the study of natural history.   The printing press facilitated the spread of the endless botanies and herbals, and the hope of finding new remedies in the vegetable world stimulated the efforts of the great botanists of the time.

This advance of science, combined with a better organization of surgical teaching, led in the latter part of the century to the appearance of a remarkable body of able surgeons in England whose writings are even now of interest and value.

The effect of the Reformation itself was complex, for while it disposed men's minds in favour of changes where needful, it drew off many of the best intellects of the time to theological controversies ; and the wholesale destruction of libraries, schools, and monasteries inflicted a gigantic loss on the nation in general and on science in particular.   It was a question whether the gilds of the barber surgeons, and even the universities themselves would not be destroyed by the plunderers of church property. Both one and the other were bound to religious observances and had in one sense a religious origin. Both were possessed of great wealth, part of which was burdened with trusts for providing services for the souls of the dead, so that there was a great temptation to destroy them. However, the powerful trade gilds, livery companies, and universities were successful in protecting themselves, and though they had to surrender the property which represented the religious trusts, they retained their power and the rest of their wealth.

The destruction of the infirmaries and hospitals was carried out with startling completeness; not only those hospitals which were almshouses for the poor and aged, but those which treated the sick were swept away. A few were refounded at once, but two centuries passed before hospitals reappeared in any numbers. Meanwhile surgery and surgical teaching were deprived of an invaluable aid.

2. The Progress of Surgery Abroad

Two subjects especially exercised the minds of surgeons in Europe at the beginning of the century. These were the effects and treatment of gunshot wounds and the question of the origin and treatment of syphilis. *Jerome of Brunswick* (1497) had taught that gunshot wounds were poisoned and caused burns, and that they required special treatment, and this opinion had many supporters. Among them was the celebrated *Vigo*, an Italian surgeon, whose *Practica Copiosa* (1514) attained immense popularity and ran through fifty-two editions. The controversy was fought out vigorously, and lasted over the whole century.

Maggi of Bologna showed by experiments in 1551 that these wounds were neither poisoned nor burned by the heat of the bullet, but still the dispute ran on, though it was pointed out that many of their peculiarities were really due to the local bruising which these low velocity projectiles caused.

Ambroise Paré, the most brilliant surgeon of the time, in his book on gunshot wounds (1545), had also denied their poisoning. We all know how he gave up the use of boiling oil for disinfecting them when the supplies accidentally ran short, and he found that they did equally well with other dressings.

Paré began life as a poor boy at Laval, and seems to have been a barber surgeon's apprentice, but got a post for two years at the Hôtel Dieu in Paris as house-surgeon. Having made the most of his opportunities, he went to the wars as a military surgeon for thirty years, and so great was his skill that he was made surgeon to the King in 1552, and under four successive monarchs he retained that office till the end of his life in 1590, beloved and trusted equally by princes and the poor. He quali- fied as a barber surgeon in 1541, and was admitted to the ranks of the surgeons of St. Côme in 1554. Like Vesalius, he had been a student of anatomy under Silvius, and, ever learning, he found time to write two books on anatomy, and one on obstetrics, besides volume after volume on surgery. He has been credited with the invention, or at least with the practical introduction, of podalic version in midwifery. Great as his work was in that respect, he will be chiefly remembered for his use of the ligature in bleeding during amputation. It was nothing new to employ ligatures for bleeding vessels, but everyone used the cautery in amputa- ting. Paré consulted with his colleagues on the subject, and thought out the matter carefully with suitable experiments, till he succeeded in showing the immense superiority of ligatures over the cruel and uncertain cauteries which destroyed the flesh and often failed to stop the bleeding, though applied again and again.

Pierre Franco (*b.* 1503) took up the scientific treatment of several branches of surgery which had been left to the hands of quacks and irregular practitioners. He reformed the operations on hernia, where it had been a common practice to remove one or both testicles. He practically created the operation for strangulated hernia, and attained great renown for his work in operating for stone and again for cataract. Indeed, he is said to be the first to perform suprapubic cystotomy.

3. The Elizabethan Surgeons in England

For the first time in our history we find a striking group of able surgeons, whose writings are still of interest. In them, too, we find the questions of the nature of gunshot wounds and syphilis ably debated.

Gale, the author of the *Encheiridion of Surgery,* 1563, the first complete work on the subject in English, wrote a volume on these gunshot wounds, showing that they were not poisoned. Both he, Halle, and Clowes are now most commonly remembered from their amusing attacks on the quacks of the time, the pretenders who had failed in other callings, the tinkers, jugglers, serving men, ignorant women, the sharpers who called on sick men as loving neighbours and recommended a surgeon, from whom they boldly claimed a percentage. Gale was a man, however, of high character, whose memorable ethical rules should not be forgotten. He lays down that the surgeon must use no deceit or guile towards his patients; must do his work courteously, gently, and cause as little pain as possible ; complete his cure as quickly as he can ; and undertake no case simply for lucre, though he should claim a proper reward for his work.   No operation may be done which is not for the real good of the patient, and no patient may be promised a cure which is impossible.

William Clowes was one of the best types of military surgeons, and is always entertaining and vigorous.   He was a Warwickshire man, and had served in the Earl of Warwick's army at Havre, and afterwards in Flanders under Leicester, and again in the navy against the Armada.   He became surgeon to Queen Elizabeth, and belonged to the staff of St. Bartholomew's Hospital.   His *Proved Practice for Young Surgeons* is chiefly a collection of cases illustrating such subjects as shot wounds, gangrene and the method of operation in gangrene, wounds of the omentum, wounds of the head, a rapier wound through the thigh complicated by syphilis, and the condition of two gentlemen who were burned by gunpowder.   He, like his contemporaries, is apt to go into endless details as to the composition of his lotions and ointments, in which he had great faith, but he was a bold and careful surgeon.   We should remember, however, that the new study of botany raised great hopes as to the value of vegetable extracts in healing wounds at this time. He was quite clear that ordinary shot wounds were not poisoned, but once he met with a case which convinced him that a bullet might be intentionally made so, and, if it were retained long enough, infect the wound. A lieutenant, a strong, vigorous man of twenty-six, was shot in the buttock. Clowes dressed the wound, but could not reach the bullet, and left him in his bed inside the fort to get a night's sleep. Violent pain, fever, and rigors came on, and as soon as the gates were opened in the morning, Clowes was hurriedly sent for. The man was terribly changed, the wound had become the colour of ashes or lead, and the limb was swollen. Clowes sent word to the commanding officers, and a consultation was held. An experienced physician advised that the wound should be freely opened up and the bullet reached or extracted at all costs with special forceps and tentacles, and that then the tissues should be scarified and a cupping glass applied over them, since the wound was undoubtedly poisoned. Clowes confessed that he had never met with a wound from a poisoned bullet, and argued that the heat of the explosion would disinfect it, saying, too, that the tissues round a shot wound were so bruised that they easily became infected from foul air. Still, he allowed that some authorities taught otherwise. However, he agreed to carry out the advice of the consultant, and succeeded in extracting the bullet, which was flattened and ragged on one side, and of a curious colour, as though rusty iron, green copperas, or some glassy substance had been sprinkled on it. When heated, these stains disappeared, but further analysis was impossible. The cupping and subsequent dressings led to a successful issue, though a violent attack of fœtid diarrhœa prostrated the patient.

To clear up this question of poisoned bullets, Clowes, when at Portsmouth, got the Master Gunner to have an arrow shot out of a musket. When this was done the feathers of the arrow were found to be unsinged by the fire. The same thing happened with a sheaf of arrows fired from a caliver. If, then, the explosion did not burn feathers, it clearly could not purify a bullet. His military friends assured him that bullets were sometimes intentionally poisoned, and to use them was punishable with death under the Law of Arms. Indeed, they had known men executed on that charge. This satisfied Clowes as to the possibility of such wounds.

One more of his cases may be narrated briefly. In 1573 a soldier named Giles was shown him, who had been wounded three years previously in Flanders by a bullet entering the left iliac fossa. There was still a deep sinus there, which was seriously affecting his health, and the situation of the bullet could not be determined. Clowes made futile efforts to reach it by long probes. He then enlarged the orifice, introduced sponge tents, and even caustics, but he was still unable to get a flexible probe down to find the bullet. He bethought himself that a liquid might penetrate, and injected through a long tube a solution containing alum and sublimated silver, leaving it in while the patient was kept in a suitable position. Twenty-three hours after, pain and swelling began in the right buttock near the anus, which was poulticed. Next day he cut down on the swelling, found the bullet there, and removed it. After a series of dressings and injections the wounds healed up completely. The question of syphilis also was of great importance in the view of Clowes. He not only translated a work by J. Almenas, the Spaniard, upon syphilis, but wrote a volume himself on the same subject, *De Morbo Gallico.*

J. Halle of Maidstone, another of this group of writers, was a scholar and a botanist who translated the *Chirurgia Parva* of Lanfranc in 1565, and wrote a textbook of anatomy, besides his *Historical Expostulation against the Beastly Abusers of Chirurgery and Physick in our Time.* He tells us that he translated Lanfranc out of " old Saxony English into our usual or vulgar phrase," and compared it with Latin, French, and other English versions.   It is interesting to find him criticizing Lanfranc for advising that "nerves" or sinews, when cut through, should be sutured, especially in children, so that the recovery of motion might be possible.   Halle, with all respect to his author, warns the reader that this is opposed by many writers, and thinks it bad surgery.   Indeed, the fear of touching nerves or tendons remained for a long time.

His notes, surgical and botanical, extend to twice the length of Lanfranc's treatise.   He frequently quotes from the Herbal of " Master Doctor Turner, our countryman," an exponent of the new science ; and we find him referring to the " crimson or grass vetch which I have growing in my garden at Maydstone," and giving accurate descriptions of native plants.   His anatomy is fairly exact, and in one place he stops to point out an important error in Gemini's plates from Vesalius, which represented the vena arteriosa as one with the aorta, and confused the work of the pulmonary artery and vein.   He intentionally refuses to enumerate the muscles, or to give their origins and insertions, though he knew that Vigo had distinguished over 500.   Indeed, his space was already taxed by the inclusion of much physiology, and the names of the bones and other organs in Latin, Greek, and English.

John Banister was a still more remarkable man
for his time. He was born in 1533 ; went to Oxford,
and took the licence in medicine, 1573 ; served as a
surgeon in the expedition to Havre with his "dear
and loving friend" William Clowes, and again in
Flanders. He lived for a time at Nottingham, but
came to London and lectured in anatomy for the
barber surgeons, 1581 ; and was admitted a member
of the company next year.   He wrote (1) a treatise
on surgery, 1575 ; (2) another treatise on anatomy,
The History of Man, 1578 ; (3) *A Compendious
Chirurgery gathered and translated especially out
of Wecker*, 1585, with copious annotations and
numerous corrections ; (4) *The Antidotary Chirurgical*, a collection of surgical formulæ.   As he
continued to live in London he obtained from the
Queen, in consequence of his military services, a
letter to the College of Physicians directing them
to license him to practise medicine in the London
area as well as surgery, which was granted with
the condition that he should obtain a consultation
with a member of the college in dangerous cases.
Sir D'Arcy Power considers this was an attempt to
further the reunion of medicine and surgery which
Clowes, Gale, and Hall had sought to effect (*Notes
on Early Portraits of John Banister, of William
Harvey, etc.*, by D'Arcy Power).   However, such
important changes had taken place that anything

like a union of the two branches was impossible then.   New and powerful corporations had been created with different interests which could not be harmonized.

4. THE ORGANIZATION OF SURGERY

At the beginning of the Tudor period there were still military surgeons and barber surgeons, though the two bodies worked amicably together, and some university physicians and surgeons.

The Military Surgeons were not united into any royal corps, but were attached to individual commanders or noblemen.   Thus John Harvey (*temp.* Henry VII.) gives us a brief sketch of the position and pay of army surgeons at the time.

" He that will be a surgeon in the wars must elect and choose him a captain of some noble, liberal man that loves his men well, and know what he will allow his surgeons a day.   If he be a nobleman that is your captain, he will allow you, as others do, two shillings [*i.e.*, about £1] a day to the chief surgeon, and the second 1s. 9d., to the third 1s. 4d., and also a groat apiece of every soldier every month. His balderic [the red sash which we can even now remember as worn by every officer, and to which the sword was formerly attached] must be of his master's colours about his neck, with a spatula before, and behind with the King's arms in like manner.   Besides [he can reckon on] the cases that he will have abroad among noblemen and other soldiers, if he be perfect in his science, and be well

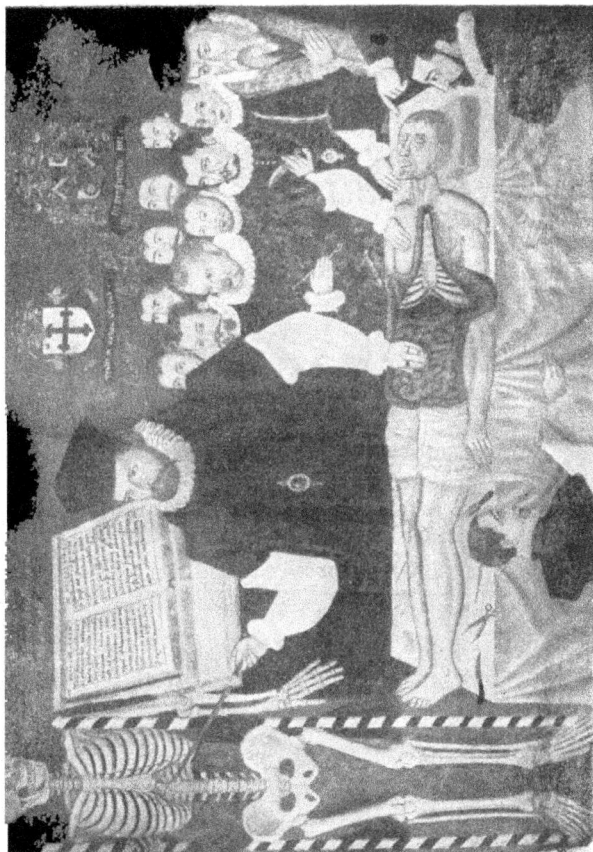

JOHN BANISTER (1533-1610)

DELIVERING THE VISCERAL LECTURE AT THE BARBER SURGEONS' HALL, LONDON, IN 1581.

From a contemporary painting now in the Hunterian Library at Glasgow.

acquainted, gentle [manly], close, honest, and merry. Also know what your master will allow unto your coffer [surgeon's chest]. Some noblemen will allow, if they are liberal, twenty nobles, some five pounds, some five marks. [The contents were supposed to be maintained by the groat from each soldier till Charles I. made a special grant.] The captain will carry your coffer, or else you must have a waggon with a horse or two amongst you, wherein you shall put your tent, your chests, your bedstead and bed, and your clothes, two or three shirts, two or three pairs of hose, your cassock or nightgown, your hood and hose of frieze, your high boots and ford boots, your various shoes, and other things necessary for a surgeon" (MS., Ashmole, *Bodleian Quarterly Record*, I.).

The army surgeon continued to be a company officer till 1665. Thus there was one surgeon to each hundred men in the army at Quentin, 1557; the surgeon's pay then given was a shilling a day in the infantry, and two shillings in the cavalry. The same rate of pay applies to surgeons of the 70,000 men raised against the Armada, and in the Irish campaigns. Gale tells us that he recruited seventy-two surgeons in London in one year for the army and navy, but that twenty years later there was a difficulty in getting men. It seems incredible that the first great military hospital was one formed in 1597 at the siege of Amiens.

The Barber Surgeons' Companies grew more

6

powerful, and under a new law no alterations could be made in their ordinances except with the assent of the Lord Chancellor, the Treasurer, and certain of the judges. The rules of the London Company thus revised in 1529 included an obligation to obtain a consultation in serious cases, another that everyone on the surgical side must attend the weekly lecture on surgery, and give a reading in his turn, or find a substitute. No one might take a patient who was under the care of another, but the patient might change his surgeon if he wished after paying the first one. Outsiders might not be admitted as members without the consent of a majority of the livery. The city ordinance of 1364 was annexed to the document laying down that the craft should be so ruled that no false work should be done in it.

The Tudor autocracy had a definitely favourable effect on the progress of medicine and surgery. There is some reason to think that Henry VIII., before he became involved in matrimonial troubles and ecclesiastical reforms, projected a complete reorganization of both arts, and he actually succeeded in carrying out a large part of this scheme.

The Act of 1511.—The first step which he took was with the aim of checking the crowd of quacks and pretenders which flourished in every part of the country. They were forbidden by the Act of 1421, and in the towns the mayor's officers could be forced to arrest them by the barber surgeons' companies; but it seems to have been no one's business in the country districts to present them before a court-leet, or at the assizes, or to summon them before a justice of the peace. Many of them, too, were sheltered by ecclesiastical immunities. The government saw that the easiest way was to impose the work on the bishops. They were already judges in church matters, and had officials to carry out their decisions. Their jurisdiction in certain matters extended not only over laymen, but over most monasteries, almshouses, and hospitals. Above all, they could compel in their visitations the churchwardens in each parish and officials in each institution to present offenders before them. Accordingly, in 1511 an Act of Parliament (3 Henry VIII.) was passed, which attained its object by giving the bishops the power to license practitioners and to punish offenders. Each bishop must have a board of examiners in medicine and surgery, and anyone who failed to pass or could not produce a satisfactory diploma was to be punished. There is no evidence that the Church had ever undertaken this work before Henry thrust it on them. The Council of Bézieres (1310) had laid down that priests and monks must get the bishop's licence before they practised surgery, but that did not concern laymen, and was only a local law. Midwives, too, had been subject to some episcopal rules, because baptism might be neglected in emergencies. There were episcopal decrees to prevent the overlaying of children by ordering all infants to have a separate bed till they were old enough to say "Lie further." The neglect of patients in hospitals, too, was a common subject of inquiry at visitations, but no instance of ecclesiastical supervision of the practice of surgery by laymen in earlier periods has been discovered.

The Act 3 Henry VIII., c. 11, recites that since physic and surgery have been and are practised by unskilled persons, such as smiths, weavers, and women, to the grievous hurt of the king's lieges, it is therefore enacted by parliament that "no person within the City of London nor within seven miles of the same shall take upon him to exercise and occupy as a physician or surgeon except he be first examined, approved, and admitted by the Bishop of London or the Dean of St. Paul's for the time being, calling to him or them four doctors of physic, and for surgery other expert persons in that faculty . . . upon the pain of forfeiture for every month that they do occupy as physicians or surgeons . . . of five pounds," half of this to be paid to the informer. Also that no person in the rest of the country shall practise as physician or surgeon unless he be licensed as above, or by the Bishop of the diocese, who shall call to him as assessors such expert persons as he shall think fit. Nothing in this Act shall be prejudicial to the Universities of Oxford and Cambridge and their privileges.

This licensing by the Bishops, based on an Act of Parliament, continued till near the end of the eighteenth century at least. It must not be confused with the power of the Archbishop of Canterbury to confer degrees, which arose from his right as Papal Legate, and exists to-day, though it gives no licence to practise. It is doubtful whether visitation inquiries as to quacks were made at first. There is a curious absence of them in the sixteenth century visitation articles printed by Frere, but the articles of the seventeenth century contain them pretty regularly. Dr. Cuthbert Atchley noted some sixty instances where the church-wardens were asked on oath what ignorant persons without a licence from a university or the ordinary had taken on themselves to practise medicine or surgery. Abbot, in 1612, asks how many physicians, chirurgeons, or midwives there were, and what were their qualifications, skill, and behaviour. In Bristol, Goodman in 1634, Laud in 1640, and Ironside in 1662 made search for unlicensed practitioners.

It does not appear that this Act interfered with the licensing powers of the barber surgeon companies, for a year later the charter of the London company was confirmed, mentioning those very powers. Nor do instances of any conflict occur for a long time. In 1599 the Bishop of London, at the request of the company, promised that no one should receive his licence to practise until he had produced evidence of passing the company's examination. The company had already, in 1555, laid down that a certificate for that purpose would only be granted after the second examination in surgery and anatomy, the Grand Diploma, had been gained. Probably, where a respectable examining body existed, the bishops refrained from calling together their board of examiners. Nearly a hundred years later (1670) in Bristol, an active Vicar-General argued that the barber surgeons' licence was invalid unless the bishop granted one too. The local company had no Royal Charter, but the corporation under whom they acted had, and their position as a co-ordinate licensing power seemed so strong that his attempt failed, though the bishop continued to grant licences both for the city of Bristol and for the county of Gloucester independently of the company.

In 1710 the Archbishop of Canterbury was

requested not to issue licences for London, because the Act 3 Henry VIII. gave the power for London only to the Bishop of London, and the Act 32 Henry VIII. confirmed the rights of the company, while the Bishop from time to time had licensed only those certified by the company. Copies of this statement were sent to the Bishops of London, Winchester, and Rochester. On another application in 1713 the Bishop of London confirmed the promise of his predecessor in 1599, and in 1715 agreed not to summon to his visitation those who had only the company's licence.

On the whole, we come to the conclusion that the Act of 1511 gave an independent licensing power to the bishops extending over the dioceses of the whole country; but this was not regarded as interfering with the powers of properly authorized barber surgeon companies for their districts, or with those of the universities. Moreover, before a man whom the bishop licensed could practise in a city he must get the freedom of that city. This was an expensive matter, costing perhaps £200 of our money, which alone would check the numbers entering through that portal; while freedom of the city to one who had been apprenticed to a member of a city company was only the equivalent of thirty-five shillings.

Henry's next step was to create a College of

Physicians, whom he endowed with ample powers, at the instigation of Linacre and others in 1518.

The licensing bodies then in London were the Universities, the Bishop, the Gilds of Surgeons and Barber Surgeons, which soon became the United Company, and the College of Physicians. With the history of the latter body we are not now concerned except as part of the general organization of the profession. The Act which completed their powers asserted the unity of medicine and surgery, or rather that the science of medicine includes surgery as one of its branches.

The Act of 1540.—We now come to the most important change in the organization of surgery which the government undertook. In 1540 parliament found time to give a permanent position by statute to the teachers of surgery in London by uniting the incorporated or chartered company of barbers and surgeons with the gild of pure or military surgeons. The new company received all the powers given under the charters of Edward IV., Henry VII., and Henry VIII., with certain additions. The Act declared that those members who practised surgery should not in future carry on barbery, and that the barbers should not undertake any surgery except dental work. The separation of the two callings was to be complete, though united under a single corporation for legal purposes. Two Masters, as before, were at the head of the surgical section, and two at the head of the barbers, who now included all who were not surgeons. The new company got the lands and the hall of the old one, together with the exemption from bearing arms and from serving on watches and inquests, though to avoid ill feeling the company afterwards agreed to waive this right, except for those who were actually practising surgery, and even these had to assist at the inquests in ward moots. It also received power, like the bishops, to punish with penalties up to £5 a month all unlicensed practitioners in London, whether natives or aliens, freemen of the city or "foreigners." Finally, the company was to have two bodies of executed criminals each year for the study of anatomy and "the better knowledge of the science or faculty of surgery."

We have already seen that long before the charter of 1462 the company had taken up educational work, and now a vigorous effort was made to improve it. There had been from an early period a reader in anatomy, usually an able physician like William Cunningham or Julius Burgaineus, but sometimes a surgeon was chosen. This official gave four groups of public lectures annually. Twice a day for three days the body was the centre of a crowd of spectators, while the reader lectured and his stewards dissected for him. Afterwards the demonstrator went over the work again with the student apprentices. Even this did not suffice for the more energetic students and teachers, who used to get permission to carry on private dissections in the theatre and to make special investigations.

On Tuesdays through a great part of the year every surgical member of the company had to attend a meeting at which a paper on surgery was read. At some periods each man took his turn in bringing forward a subject, but the rule varied, and at others a selected surgeon or doctor of physic gave a course of surgical lectures. This was the origin of the Gale and other annual lectures.

The examiners in surgery presided over the examination of the students who had served their apprenticeship. Each apprentice in 1555, after passing his first examination in surgery and anatomy, received a temporary licence, and his progress was then tested every six months till he was thought fit to be admitted to the Grand Diploma as a master in Surgery and Anatomy, and not until then might he apply for the bishop's seal or licence. Exhibitions (Young, pp. 183, 187) were given to some promising students to study at the universities, and in 1566 we find the company sending a man to Magdalene College, Cambridge,

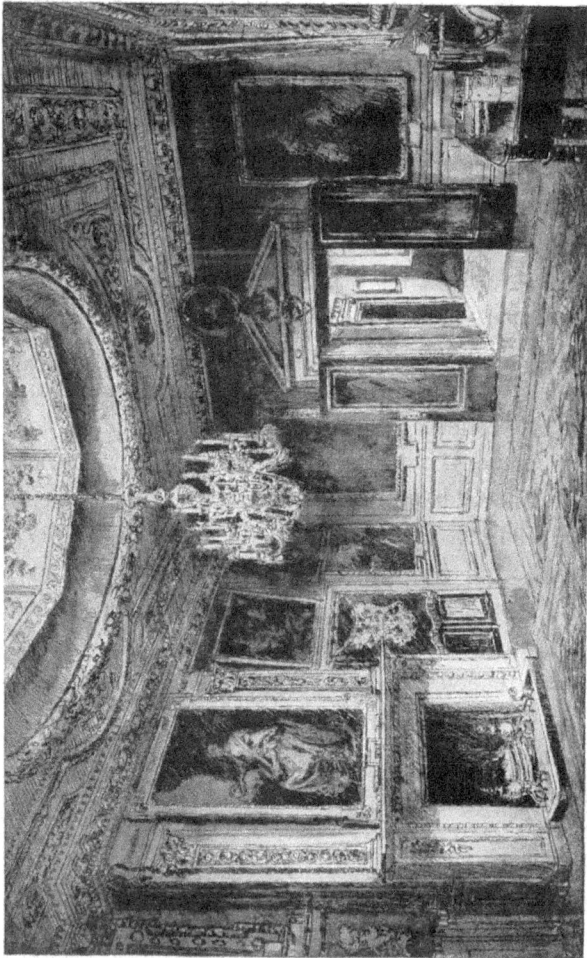

COURT ROOM, BARBER SURGEONS' HALL.

From a drawing by Hanslip Fletcher, by permission of the Worshipful Company of Barbers.

to complete his studies in medicine and surgery, on
the understanding that he would act as tutor afterwards at the Barbers' Hall. If a man had not been
apprenticed under the company, and wished to
practise in London, he had usually to produce his
indentures, then pass the examination, and join the
company as a " Foreign Brother."   Sea surgeons
became Foreign Brothers under special rules, as
they could not attend the necessary meetings and
lectures, and many surgeons living elsewhere
became Foreign Brothers for the sake of the
diploma. Occasionally a specialist was thus licensed
—e.g., Thomas Blackburn, a gynæcologist and
accoucheur in 1611.

We may add that of all the thirty-nine livery
companies of London the so-called Barber Surgeons
were the most numerous.   In 1537 they had 185
members, while the Skinners had 151, the Haber-
dashers 120, the Fishmongers 109, and the
Merchant Tailors 96.

Thus the Act of 1540 succeeded in creating for
London an active educational and licensing body.
Its high standard of efficiency influenced the
companies in other cities.   In York the company
appears to have applied to London to find them
two teachers of anatomy in 1555, and their new
ordinances in 1592 insist on the examination of all
new practitioners coming into the city, as well as

of apprentices when they had finished their term, under ample penalties. In Norwich the physicians in some way joined the old barber surgeon gild, and a compulsory lecture every three weeks was provided for under a scheme of 1561, but we know little of the results. The Dublin chartered gild was united by Elizabeth in 1572, with an existing society of surgeons on the London model, and for a time even the arms of the London company were used by the Irish body. The surgeons and barbers of Edinburgh received, under a charter from James IV. in 1506, the monopoly of practice, and the right to the body of one criminal after execution for anatomical purposes annually. It was laid down that no one should practise surgery until he had been diligently examined and tested, especially in anatomy and " in the nature and complexion of every member of man's body." No apprentice might be taken until he could read and write. No barber should practise surgery unless expert and knowing fully the things mentioned above. We must not omit to mention one extra-ordinary grant they received—viz., a monopoly of the manufacture and sale of alcohol, which is the more singular as they do not seem to have included apothecaries in their ranks. The right of exemption from bearing arms and from serving on juries was given them by Queen Mary on condition that they paid their taxes and gave medical service in time of war to the armies.

In Aberdeen the gild was incorporated by the town council in 1537.

5. ANATOMY

The century is particularly wonderful for the outburst of interest in anatomy, greater, perhaps, than in any other period. The study had been slowly growing, with few great discoveries, in spite of the public dissections at various universities which had gone on for two centuries. In the great artists of the Renaissance exact and truthful representations of the body became the rule, but it needed the vigour and eloquence of Vesalius the Belgian, a pupil of Jaques Sylvius at Paris, and afterwards lecturer at Padua, to make men see that the accepted anatomy of the time was full of errors. With infinite labour he brought together the true facts in his great work *De Fabricâ Humani Corporis*, 1543, a book "which revolutionized an entire science" and overthrew the hoary errors of classical anatomy. Fired by his success, Fallopius, Servetus, Eustachius, Variolus, and many others struggled on during the next thirty years to complete the outlines he had sketched, and with such success that their names, given to the organs they discovered, still meet the student at every turn, like Arctic islands

named from early travellers.   Anatomy became
one of the most popular studies of the day, and the
new facts which were elucidated in a short period
seem endless.   In England, though the great name
of Vicary for a time popularized a new edition of
an ancient anatomy, *The Anatomy of Man's Body*,
the teaching of the Italian school rapidly became
known through numerous lecturers in the universities and great cities.   The leader of the movement
was John Caius of Norwich, who had formerly
settled in Padua as Professor of Greek.   Whilst
there he was a lodger in the same house as Vesalius
himself, and imbibed his enthusiasm for anatomy.
After returning to England in 1541 he lectured on
it in London and Cambridge, arousing widespread
interest.   Thomas Gemini brought out in 1545 in
London copper-plate illustrations of Vesalius's work,
and when Caius came into power at Cambridge he
made provision in the statutes of his remodelled
college, Gonville and Caius, for yearly dissections
(1557). It was in keeping with Caius's character that
after inaugurating this movement he ordained that
the bodies dissected should be treated with respect,
and afterwards buried solemnly by the whole
college with as much reverence and order as if they
had been the bodies of worthy persons.   Besides
lecturing and organizing the medical school in his
college, Caius spent some of the later years of his

life in bringing out editions of Hippocrates and
Galen with comments. The Edwardian statutes
of the two universities had made anatomy compulsory for all students of medicine and surgery, and
the Regius Professor at Cambridge had to "make
one anatomy" every year if desired. Among
the students attracted to Caius College was
William Harvey in 1594, who went on to Padua
to work under Fabricius, and soon utilized his
anatomical studies for his great discoveries on the
circulation of the blood (*A History of the Study of
Anatomy in Cambridge*, by Alex. Macalister, F.R.S.).

J. Halle's treatise was an improvement on Vicary,
but, after all, a mere students' handbook. Banister
seems to have had a higher aim in his *History of
Man*, 1578. A charmingly realistic picture has
recently been reproduced and described by Sir
D'Arcy Power, which shows Banister conducting
an anatomy lecture in the Barber Surgeons' Hall in
1581, with a volume of *Realdus Columbus* open
by him as his textbook. In the Netherlands this
enthusiasm for anatomy is shown to us in many
paintings of the Dutch school by De Keyser,
Nierevelt, Rembrandt, and others, with actual
portraits of the surgeons of the time grouped round
pallid corpses. In France Paré popularized the new
teaching by two treatises in French, with illustrations taken from Vesalius.   In every great city it

burgh, 1592, and at Dublin by the charter of
Elizabeth in 1593. Abroad the university movement
still showed considerable activity, not less than
twelve or fourteen new ones being founded, among
which was Leyden, a place destined to take a high
rank in medical studies. Englishmen still went
for surgical teaching to Bologna, Padua, Pisa, Paris,
Berne, Basel, and Montpellier. Caius and Harvey
both studied in Italy, as we have seen.

7. THE HOSPITALS

The hospitals of the time fell under a cloud
which was perhaps the greatest hindrance to the
advance of surgery. After the skill and wealth
which had been lavished upon them in the fifteenth
and earlier centuries they became involved in the
sequestrations of the Reformation and simply
disappeared wholesale. The London citizens found
their sick thrown into the streets without any
provision for their treatment, and the same thing
occurred all over the country. One or two insurrec-
tions arose in consequence and were sternly re-
pressed, but the Londoners approached Henry VIII.
with a scheme to lessen the scandal, offering to
find funds if he would hand over to them two or
three of the old hospitals. He accordingly refounded St. Bartholomew's seven years after its
dissolution in 1537, and later on, seeing the efforts

the citizens made, he returned the greater part of
its revenues for the relief of " the poor, aged, sick,
low, and impotent people," who were annoying His
Grace's loving subjects by begging and infecting
them with "divers great and horrible sicknesses
and diseases." His own surgeon, Thomas Vicary,
born about 1495, took a keen interest in the revived
hospital, and in 1548 accepted the post of Resident
Surgical Governor, with three surgeons under him.
This office he retained till his death in 1561 or 1562.
Vicary's support was of great value as that of a
recognized leader of the profession. He had himself
risen from the lowly position of a practitioner in
a small way at Maidstone, but went to the
metropolis, was admitted to the barber surgeon
company, and became Senior Warden in 1528, when
he was also appointed one of the Royal Surgeons.
Two years later he was made Master of the company,
and in 1535 chief surgeon to the King, with a
grant of abbey lands. In 1541 he was elected
Master of the united societies. He wrote little,
but continued to hold his office at Court under
Edward VI., Mary, and Elizabeth, as well as his
beloved hospital. At his death he left his copy of
Guy de Chauliac to the barber surgeon company.

Besides this hospital of St. Bartholomew, with
its hundred beds, St. Thomas's and the asylum of

St. Mary of Bethlehem for the insane were with
difficulty preserved in London. Elsewhere in the
country it was hopeless, if not dangerous, to attempt
to restore the hospitals. For instance, in Bristol,
Henry gave the revenues of one or two to his
physician, Dr. George Owen. Though Owen did
not dare to restore them at once to a city
which had not a hospital left, he satisfied his
conscience by handing them over after the king's
death for almshouses to the corporation, which
still derives £1,500 a year from that source. An
amusing attempt to throw the blame for the
public distress on to the surgeons and to meet
the outcry against the active suppression of quacks
is seen in the Act 34 and 35 Henry VIII. This
was in 1542, just after the dissolution and the new
incorporation of the barber surgeons. It says that,
whereas the act of 1511 had restricted practice to
properly qualified persons, since then the company
of surgeons, minding only their own lucre, have
sued kind people who have given herbs, etc., to people
with common ailments, and have not taken anything
for their pains, but have done so only for pity and
charity; whilst the licensed surgeons have taken
too high fees and let many folk rot and die; and
since many surgeons are ignorant of their work
and actually harm their patients, wherefore it is
enacted that any subject of the king having

knowledge of roots, herbs, and waters may cure
outside sores by herbs or by giving drinks for the
stone, the strangury, or for agues, without being
sued under that act. There is nothing, however,
to show whether only gratuitous practice was
allowed, and in any case the powers of the company
were confirmed by later acts without reference to
this one, and afterwards the apothecaries received
similar exclusive rights.

CHAPTER IV

1600 TO 1700 A.D.

1. THE GROWTH OF SURGERY AT HOME AND ABROAD

THERE is a curious lack of surgeons of the first rank in Europe during this century. Germany has boasted much of the fame of Fabry of Hilden, but she produced hardly anyone else, being, in fact, exhausted by the miserable Thirty Years' War. Italy is represented only by Magiati; and France, after the death of Paré, produced hardly anyone of importance.

Fabry of Hilden, near Dusseldorf (1560-1634), became the city surgeon at Berne, where he had a small hospital under his control, and published his *Six Hundred Surgical Cases and Observations.* As a military surgeon in the Thirty Years' War he attained great renown, and devised the earliest form of tourniquet. He showed that an operation on a gangrened limb, to be successful, must be made through healthy tissue. His boldness led him to attempt, successfully, operations which had previously been looked on as impossible; he made more perfect the methods for amputation of the thigh, and his clinical teaching is not his least claim to remembrance.

In Britain, where the system of education was good, in spite of the failure of the universities and the absence of hospitals, we find the survivors of the great Elizabethan surgeons, and then Wiseman, with lesser lights such as Cooke, Read, and Woodall. The last represents a new type, the naval surgeon, who became prominent as England threw herself into the struggle for the New World and traded in tropical and Eastern waters. As the country became more and more isolated from the universities of the Continent, except for the school at Leyden, she had to rely more and more on the teaching organized by the barber surgeon companies, and, good as this was, the art did not attract many brilliant men after the end of the Civil Wars and the death of Wiseman. The chief interests of educated men of the time centred rather in the subsidiary sciences—anatomy, physiology, chemistry, mathematics, physics, and botany—which made gigantic progress, but as yet could not, in most instances, be helpful to surgery itself. That change did not come for more than a century—*i.e.*, until Hunter and his followers began to think as men of science as well as perfectly skilled artists in surgery.

It is a curious fact that the advances in these new sciences were largely made outside the universities, in small societies or academies all over Europe. One brilliant exception exists. Anatomy, physics, and mathematics were taken up with vigour and enthusiasm at Cambridge, as the names of Isaac Newton, Glisson, and their followers remind us, but the rule remains that, for the future, the chief researches in natural science were fostered by small bodies of advanced students periodically meeting for the purpose. The discoverer did not any longer read his paper before an assembled university, but at a meeting of his own special academy or society. These little academies then sprang up all over Europe, like the universities did in the twelfth century. The first of them appeared as long ago as 1560 at Naples, and was named Porta's Academy ; the society of the Lynxes at Rome followed in 1607 ; the Cimenti at Florence, 1657 ; the Académie des Sciences at Paris, 1665 ; and the Gesellschaft Naturforschender Aertze, 1652, and many others arose in succession. In England the Royal Society, which had begun at Oxford during the war, was incorporated in 1662, and united the most able men of the time in scientific studies. Of this opportunity physiologists and chemists quickly availed themselves, and even surgeons from time to time brought forward the results of their observations. We have here, then, the forerunners of the medical and surgical societies which in the nineteenth century were to take such a large part in aiding post-graduate study. The barber surgeons had insisted on frequent meetings for scientific discussion, and we find Glisson threshing out the difficulties of rickets at the sessions of a medical society, but notices of any surgical society or debate are probably unknown before the middle of the eighteenth century.

2. The Chief English Surgeons

The first half of the century was not prolific in great names. Bulleine, Read, Scarborough, Woodall, Cooke, and Wiseman may be mentioned.

Alexander Read, M.D., was, like Banister, one of the few who realized the ideal union of medicine and surgery, for he was both a Fellow of the Royal College of Physicians and a (foreign) brother and lecturer of the barber chirurgeons. His " Treatise of the first part of Surgery called by me Συνθετικὴ, the part which teacheth the reunition of the parts of the body disjoined, containing the methodical doctrine of wounds delivered in lectures in the Barber Chirurgeons' Hall upon Tuesdays appointed for these exercises and the keeping of their courts," was published in 1638. He had been educated at Aberdeen, had studied surgery also in France, and is a clear, exact, and learned writer. The substance of his lectures is carefully arranged. Thus the students are to observe so many things as to the wound itself, so many as to the state of the patient, and certain others as to the proper treatment. A wound, he says, is a solution of continuity caused by an external instrument. The reunition is produced by (1) agglutination in the case of those healed by first intention, where no middle substance intervenes; by (2) concarnation in others. To bring about the first, the lips of the wound are to be brought together gently and by degrees, not stretching one more than another. If stiff from exposure, they must be fomented; the superficial parts must exactly fit together, and the deep parts or inner sides also. No pledget must be left between them. Wounds must be held together by (1) dry stitching—*i.e.*, by strips of cloth or plaster glued to the flesh near and their free edges drawn together by threads; by (2) bandaging; or by (3) stitching with needles. This latter method includes the continuous or glover's stitch, as in wounds of the bowels, the non-continuous, and the gastroraphia, for wounds of the abdomen where "the peritoneum, being a membrane, would not consolidate without the intercourse of flesh." In some cases the needles are left in the wound and the thread twisted around them, as in hare-lip and

wounds of the trachea arteria. Quite occasionally
he allows himself a digression, as in his discussion
of the nature of pain, and, again, after laying
down that *the spleen may be excised without harm*,
he describes his great experimental excision on
a dog. This operation was one which

"Master Gillam and I made in Dr. Bonham's
house. First an incision was made in the left side
hard under the short ribs four inches in length
through all the containing parts of the abdomen.
Then the spleen was drawn out. Thirdly, all the
vessels by which it was bound to the adjacent and
contiguous parts we bound to prevent the im-
moderate flux of blood. Fourthly, we cut away
the spleen near to the substance of it. Fifthly, we
stitched the parts of the abdomen and left the
healing of the parts to nature. All the wounded
parts were in a short time healed, but about six
weeks afterwards the cur was mangy, the spleen
belike not drawing into it the feculent blood"
(p. 231).

This was perhaps the first excision of the spleen
performed in this country.

As to the old question of gunshot wounds, he
lays down (1) that they are not poisonous if nothing
be added to the bullet in the making, for lead, gunpowder, and the materials of the powder are harmless;
(2) that such wounds always present much contu-
sion and injury of surrounding parts; (3) that a
bullet may be made to absorb poison which will

not be driven out by the heat of the explosion, and if such a bullet be retained it may poison a wound (p. 108).

He recognized some seven methods of stopping hæmorrhage : (1) Pledgets of lint moistened with white of egg or vinegar and water. (2) Ligation of the bleeding vessel, whether artery or vein, when large vessels are wounded, care being taken not to include a nerve in the ligature and not to tie it too tight lest the silk or hemp used cut through the coats and lead to fresh bleeding. He thinks, however, that Ambroise Paré's advice to use ligatures in amputations is wrong. (3) The transverse section of the bleeding vessel, which should be lifted up by a hook and twisted after division. (4) The actual cautery or escharotics. (5) Incarnative medicaments, such as aloes, comfrey, frankincense, or equisetum. (6) Opening a vein on the opposite side of the body while bandages are applied to the extremities. (7) The application of cold to the whole body, or a large dose of opium, especially in epistaxis.

We may conclude with a little story in his own words, showing the value of caustics, and still more his resourcefulness in difficulties :

"About twenty years ago, returning from the Bath in Somersetshire to the Holt, about five miles from Chester, where then I remained, having lodged in Newport in Shropshire by the way, I

was called by this Lord Gerard's grandfather to
Gerard's Bramley to take a view of his tailor, who
had fractured both the facils of the leg a little
below the knee about the breadth of a palm.
When I did behold the fracture, with a wound, and
the extenuation of the body (for the accident fell
out ten weeks before), neither were the bones
united, and, besides, there was a great tumour in
the knee, I pronounced a lingering death to the
party unless he were out of hand dismembered
above the knee. Being entreated by the sick party
and the Earl to perform the operation, I yielded
unto their request ; but having by me neither instrument nor medicament, I supplied the place of both.
I made a medicament with umber and unslaked
lime, taking equal parts of each, which I found
there (the house then being in reparation). I used
a joiner's tooth saw, newly toothed, and in the
presence of two chirurgeons, Messrs. S. and D., I dismembered the Lord's tailor (unto whom the Lord
gave £10 a year during his lifetime, who lived many
years afterwards). When I dressed the wound the
fourth day I found the mouths of all the vessels shut
by incarnation, so powerful was the restrictive medicament made by equal parts of umber and unslaked
lime reduced to the form of a liniment by the
addition of whites of eggs beaten and the hair of a
hare."

John Woodall, 1569-1643, the Surgeon-General
to the East India Company, served in Willoughby's
expedition to France, and spent eight years travelling in Germany, Poland, and France. He was
one of the surgeons at St. Bartholomew's Hospital,

and describes many of his cases there. We find him Master of the barber surgeons in 1633, and later on as one of the examiners. Once more in his life he was ordered on military service to treat the wounded from the fighting at the Isle of Ré in 1627.

Among his writings is the *Surgeon's Mate*, containing full accounts of the surgical instruments in use, the dressings and medicines to be provided, the treatment of wounds, abscesses, dislocations, and the method of amputations. To this he adds long accounts of scurvy, calentures, and dysentery, as necessary for the naval surgeon. He has been spoken of as the discoverer of lime and lemon juice as the remedy for scurvy, but as a matter of fact he refers to it as an established practice to send out a quantity in every ship for the purpose, and adds : "The use of the juice of lemons is a precious medicine and well tried; being sound and good [practice], let it have the chief place." He praises also watercress, wormwood, citrons, tamarinds, and even sulphuric acid lemonade.

In the *Viaticum* he concerns himself with the treatment of gunshot wounds. "The most notable difference I have ever observed," he says, "between wounds made with gunshot and other contused wounds is only a furtive hæmorrhage and a dangerous disposition to gangrene." He wrote, too, a *Treatise on the Plague*, which broke out in

England more than once during his life, and from which he had himself suffered; and another on *Gangrene*, where he argues in favour of operating in certain cases in the affected tissues, though he confesses it is contrary to the teaching of the best writers.

Two men whose practice had been largely amongst the soldiers in the Civil War have left us treatises on the surgery of the time. These are the Puritan Cooke, and Wiseman the Cavalier surgeon to Charles II. We would not willingly be without either picture of suffering humanity in the great war.

James Cooke, who had a good general practice, lived at Warwick, and published two works, *The Mellificium or Marrow of Surgery*, which became a favourite textbook for surgery, midwifery, and therapeutics; and the *Supplementum Mellificii*, a treatise on fevers, and rickets just then made fashionable by Glisson. This latter happens to be one of the rarest volumes in English medicine, and its style is not without eloquence.

Thus in discussing prosaically what is needed for the surgeon's chest for the preservation of the wounded, and the care required in its use, he continues:

" For the subject to be dealt withal is not a beast, but man, for whom in some sense the Son of God has shed His most precious blood, and

if there be neglect, it must be answered before the
Lord at the dreadful day, for blood-guiltiness in
neglecting thy duty, or for both that and drunken-
ness [leading] to the ruin of men bearing perhaps a
fuller representation of God on them than you
yourself."

Cooke is the editor or translator of the *Select
Observations on English Bodies*, by his neighbour
Dr. J. Hall, the husband of Shakespeare's daughter,
who, by the way, is accused of destroying Shakespeare's manuscripts. Cooke's interview with Mrs.
Hall at Stratford, when she showed him papers belonging to her late husband, has become famous, for
he says: "I, being acquainted with Mr. Hall's hand,
told her that one or two were her husband's, and
showed them to her. She denied it. I affirmed it
till I perceived she began to be offended." Mrs. Hall
had stated that the whole pile had been given to her
husband as security for a loan. However, Cooke
gave her the money she asked for them, took
possession of the papers, and published Hall's
Observations, which are chiefly of interest as giving
details of Shakespeare's family and friends.

The incident has been used absurdly by
Baconians to prove that Shakespeare's daughter
could not read or write, though her signature to a
deed is still extant, and her epitaph speaks of her as
witty above her sex.

The *Marrow of Surgery* is not a brilliant book,

but Cooke is at his best in describing cases he met with. In the case of a wound of the lung, he tells us how two cavalry patrols mistook each other for the enemy near Kineton, and one of them got three bullets through his chest, so that the air hissed in and out as he breathed. He was carried some ten miles to Warwick in a cart, but Cooke wisely refrained from interference with the wound, and he recovered without a check. He is rather proud of a case where he diagnosed that the heart was wounded, which he confirmed by a post-mortem. It was in a poor officer's servant, who begged a soldier of the Scottish army, when passing by, not to interfere with one of their sentries. The man savagely turned on him and stabbed him in the side with his dirk. Cooke, standing at the old gate of Warwick Castle, saw the man ride up blanched and breathless, and put him into bed, but decided that the case was hopeless, since definite signs of an injury of the heart were present, and die he did in two days or less, but in a pious and edifying manner. Whereupon Cooke verified his opinion by an examination of the corpse.

Richard Wiseman, 1620-1676, has been called the father of English surgery. The greater part of his life was spent in military and naval service, first in the Dutch navy during the Spanish war. Then he joined the Cavalier army in the west of England, where he was attached to the Prince of Wales's personal staff, and when the contest was hopeless he went into exile with him. When Charles landed again in Scotland, Wiseman again went through the campaign with him till the final defeat at Worcester, 1652. He was captured, and then set free by the Parliamentary rulers, and having obtained the barber surgeon diploma, settled down to practise in the Old Bailey. He next got thrown into the Tower for a supposed participation in a plot. He was released after a time, and served for three years in the Spanish navy. At the Restoration he became sergeant-surgeon to the King. He employed his repose in writing his classical *Treatises on Surgery*, transcribing the notes of 600 of the cases he had treated, and deducing from them, in a previously unattempted way great general principles of surgical treatment, which rendered his work the most brilliant achievement produced by English surgery up to that time. In the pages of his discourse we get glimpses by the way of the life of the combatants, the treatment of the wounded, and the course of the wars. There are cases of men wounded in sea-fights, or stabbed by savage Dunkirk or Dutch seamen, others wounded at the siege of Weymouth, or in the fight at Worcester, as well as accidents from the crowded London streets. Vivid pictures all of them, apart from the surgical lesson which he draws from each. We see at the siege of Taunton a poor soldier who had the greater part of his face, with the eyes and nose and jaw, blown away, and was left for dead among other corpses in an empty house, and afterwards found standing leaning over the half-door sightless and speechless, even the brain oozing out through the scalp wounds. It appeared that he suffered from thirst, but it was difficult to feed him. However, the wretched sufferer himself held down the root of his tongue, and poured the milk they brought him down the opening into his throat, holding his head backwards, and got down more than a quart. After that, Wiseman bound up his wounds, laid him on fresh straw, and for a week he was dressed with fomentations daily. But they had to retreat and leave the still living man behind. Again he shows us another man at Melcomb Regis who had part of the skull and brain crushed by a shot, and after the bones and flesh were pulled out of the brain substance and the wound dressed he lived seventeen days and walked a long distance, but became convulsed and died.

"I could tell you of many more wounded in the brain," he says, "but these may serve to prove what I would demonstrate—that the brain is of itself insensible, that the symptoms proceed from the pain which the meninges, etc., suffer." The vomiting, stupor, or paralyses come on when these coverings are irritated by spicules of bone or foreign bodies, or compressed by extravasated blood or depressed fractures. Even if the brain oozes out no symptoms appear, he adds, till it becomes corrupt or septic, when convulsions, " howling," and the death of the patient follow.

Though a water-drinker himself, he warns the surgeon not to cut off too suddenly all stimulants in the case of hard drinkers. His Dunkirk men were extraordinary drinkers, and " I could scarce ever cure any of them without allowing them wine." His own health failed under the hardships of his life. Again and again hæmoptysis came on, even when he was operating, but he survived for sixteen years after the Restoration to complete his chirurgical works and to enjoy his well-earned honours.

John Locke, the philosopher, author of the famous *Essay on the Human Understanding*, the close friend of Sydenham and of Isaac Newton, was also a general practitioner, though a man of considerable wealth and a student of Christ Church, Oxford. He was the Commissioner of Trade and Plantations—*i.e.*, a Colonial Minister under Charles II.— and wrote, too, on sanitary and poor law reform. A celebrated case of his may be mentioned. He opened a hydatid cyst of the liver, the patient being Lord Ashley, and maintained permanent

drainage by a silver tube which Ashley wore for
a long time.

3. THE ORGANIZATION OF SURGERY

The study and teaching of surgery was no longer
left to chance.   It was still unfortunately separated
from medicine, it was almost entirely without the
assistance which great hospitals can give, but it
was daily receiving more and more inspiration, if
not help, from the rapidly growing sciences of
anatomy, physiology, chemistry, and physics ; while
the education of the surgeon himself was carefully
carried out by two groups of corporations, the
companies of barber surgeons and the universities.

The barber surgeon companies were now at the
height of their activity, and in London, York,
Newcastle, Bristol, Norwich, Edinburgh, Glasgow,
and Dublin, students were not only apprenticed,
but went through a regular course of anatomy with
dissections, surgical lectures, and examinations,
with in many instances post-graduate work and
lectures.   Libraries were acquired by the companies, and we find in 1604 Mr. Fenton presenting
500 copies of the *Tables of Surgery* to the London
company for distribution to the members of their
surgical division.   Gale and Arris founded their
annual lectures in 1643 and 1698.   The Newcastle
company were proud of having received a copy of

were ordered to impress surgeons for the campaign at Rochelle in 1626, and for the Isle of Ré in 1627, again in 1628, and for the Scottish war in 1639, when they shipped twenty-three men to serve with the army at Newcastle. They had to find others for the Parliamentary forces in 1644, and twenty more, with their assistants, for the Dutch war in 1672. It is curious to see how history repeats itself, and how the Central War Committee of 1915 has taken the place of the company in recruiting for the army. The pay of the army surgeons under Charles I. rose to 2s. 6d. a day, and for naval surgeons 1s., with a free chest of stores on joining, and twopence a month from each soldier's pay to provide dressings and medicines. Besides the regimental surgeons, who date from 1655 (previously each company had its surgeon), there were staff surgeons, and one or more surgeons-general and physicians-general. Field hospitals, clearing stations, and base hospitals, are found in the Irish campaigns of William III. Among the military hospitals we find St. Bartholomew's, St. Thomas's, the Savoy, and Ely House, used as base hospitals, as well as Heriot House in Edinburgh, while Bath became a convalescent home for 220 men in 1652. Under the care of Marlborough, military hospitals became efficient, and were staffed by both male and female nurses.

The regimental pay of surgeons rose to 4s. a day after the Restoration, with an allowance for each company of £6 per annum for dressings and medicines.

Woodall's *Viaticum* is a mine of information as to the naval surgeon's work, instruments, drugs, and dressings.

In Scotland, the Edinburgh Corporation of the crafts of surgeons and barbers (see p. 92) obtained a new charter in 1613, and, finally, Acts of Parliament in 1641 and 1643, empowering them to arrest and fine all persons practising surgery who were not members, and defining surgery as "operations and applications upon the living and dead bodies of men, women, and children, and the curing of diseases, such as tumours, wounds, ulcers, luxations, and fractures, the curing of verolls, etc." For a great part of the century the surgeons were supreme, and oppressed the unfortunate barbers, who maintained a helpless position as a subordinate branch of the gild.

It appears that the surgeons took measures in 1648 and 1649 to exclude all barbers except those who passed an examination in surgery. This made it impossible to get a sufficient number of barbers for the town, and the town council had to step in and force them to admit a certain number. In 1695 the Corporation of Surgeons, as they then advice to the poor, and apparently to hold what corresponded to a coroner's inquest when necessary.

In 1602 the faculty laid down that surgeons must serve a seven years' apprenticeship, and then pass an examination, which included written questions, clinical cases, and a *vivâ voce*. After this the candidate had to obtain the freedom of the burgh, and was then admitted to practise. In 1617 the "Visitor or one of the Quartermasters had to teach medicine, surgery, and pharmacy to the apprentices, and to any master who liked to attend." It was also enacted that "the barbers' art being a pendicle of surgery," the barbers should pay certain fees, and not attempt surgery proper; that is, they were admitted to certain rights as a matter of grace—namely, "to be free of their own calling, and not meddle with anything else." As a rule the barber was allowed to draw teeth, let blood, and cure simple wounds, and occasionally was permitted to treat simple fractures.

Thus we get a Faculty of Physicians and Surgeons, with licensing powers and some teaching functions, for a large area in the south-west of Scotland, while the apothecaries and barber surgeons were regulated and governed by the same body. However, circumstances and the example of the British system were too strong for Lowe. The barbers of Glasgow formed a little gild of their

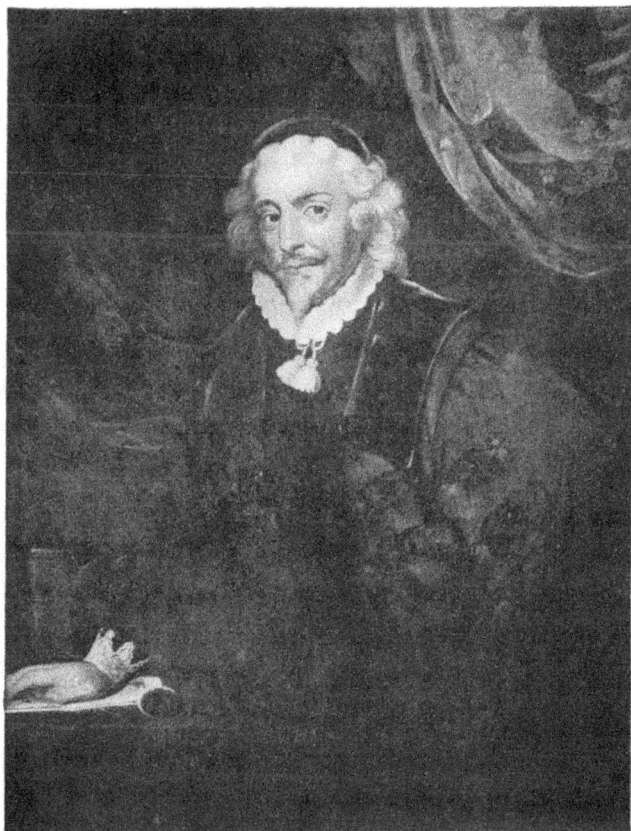

MAISTER PETER LOWE.

From a painting, by kind permission of Dr. Freeland Fergus, President of the Faculty
of Physicians and Surgeons in Glasgow.

own, and in 1656 they obtained from the corporation of their burgh " a letter of deaconry" or charter
uniting them and the chirurgeons into a gild.
This laid down in the usual way that no one should
take a cure out of another man's hand until he be
paid for his work.   The Visitor and Quartermasters
were, however, authorized to take away patients
from anyone not qualified to treat them, and to hand
them over to a more skilled person.   Since the new
gild was one of those recognized by the city, the
barbers were raised nearer to an equality with the
surgeons, and the city itself was drawn in to put
down unlicensed practice.   Of course, this arrangement was confined to the bounds of the city.   The
situation became very complex, for there was the
Faculty of Physicians and Surgeons, with licensing
powers over a wide district, recognized, too, by an
Act of Parliament in 1672, and a gild of surgeons
and barbers backed by the corporation of Glasgow.
The faculty in 1679 obtained a decision from the
law courts against the claim of the city corporation to license surgeons to practise, but the two
societies existed side by side for the rest of the
century.

4. THE HOSPITAL SCHOOLS

A curious quarrel arose in London in 1695 which
showed the rising activity of the surgeons who were
attached to the few remaining hospitals, and the

existence of hospital schools.   The London company complained that the surgeons at St. Thomas's hospital pretended to qualify persons in six months or a year, and that even one of the chief surgeons of that hospital had no qualification but what was spurious and of this sort (South, *Craft of Surgery*). The surgeons in their formal reply said that they took no apprentice for less than seven years, but that they did allow other men's apprentices or such as had served country surgeons to dress for them. They will henceforth insist on good certificates of their previous work and that security be given that such persons shall not practise in London except when admitted by the company.   Thus for the time the company maintained their authority over one of the hospital schools which were soon to rise to such importance.   This use of the hospitals as places of clinical instruction had become fashionable in some of the Italian cities and also under Von Hilden in Berne, as well as at Leyden under Van Hemne and Sylvius.

In England the practice could not at first be common from the entire absence of hospitals except the two or three which had survived the Tudor devastations.   However, it is clear that at St. Bartholomew's in 1662 students were attending the practice at the hospital, and in 1667 a library was formed there "for the use of the Governors'

young university scholars." The astonishing thing
is that, so far as is known, it had not been recognized
in early times as a regular and invaluable aid in
teaching medicine and surgery. Why did it arise
now? Was it the influence and example of the
other scientific studies, anatomy, physics, and
chemistry, which flourished at this time, leading
men to practical work instead of relying on books
and lectures?

5. THE UNIVERSITIES

On the Continent Paris, Montpellier, and Padua,
continued to be flourishing medical schools, and
Berne and still more Leyden took a high place.
We have mentioned already the introduction of
hospital clinical teaching at Berne, Leyden, and in
some of the Italian schools. Paris was still
damaged by the triangular quarrel between the
physicians, the surgical college of St. Côme, and
the barber surgeons.

The English universities showed at least one
outbreak of activity, the enthusiastic development
of anatomy and physiology at Cambridge, but
except for this the surgical and medical teaching
was at a low ebb. The Oxford Laudian statutes of
1636, tit. ix., sect. ix., §§ 4, 7, 8, as to the licence in
surgery, lay down again the two courses of anatomy,
the three " curationes " at the least, and seven

whole years' practice and study in that art (an apprenticeship), and a written approval by the Regius Professor or three other resident Doctors of Medicine. This licence gave a perpetual right to practise anywhere throughout the kingdom of England, on condition that the licentiate treated gratuitously *quatuor saltem pauperes quam primum sese occasio tulerit cum ab ipsis requisitus ;* that he would not practise medicine ; and that he would not charge too high fees, or delay a cure for the sake of gain, under pain of forfeiture of the licence. Similar rules were laid down for the licence in medicine. These licences did not attract many candidates, and, indeed, the opportunities for clinical study at the university were very small. Wood tells us that Thomas Trapham took out the licence in 1633. He became a Parliamentary army surgeon, and embalmed Charles I. and sewed on his head after his execution.

Another licentiate was the extraordinary John Pantæus, an Italian physician, who obtained the licence in 1649, and died after the Restoration at Salisbury.

In Scotland, Aberdeen University was the first to undertake medical education. From the opening of King's College, 1505, some teaching had been given by the Mediciner, but about 1630 Gordon, who then held the office, appealed to the Privy

Council for subjects for anatomy, which the local municipalities were ordered to supply to the medical school.

6. ANATOMY AND PHYSIOLOGY

The progress made in this century in these and kindred subjects was marvellous, and at no epoch have so many discoveries been crowded into so short a time. The real circulation of the blood, the use of the lymphatics, the structure of the brain, the delineation of the nervous system, the true meaning of respiration, and the minute structure of the tissues now first shown by the microscope, represent only a part of the field which was laid bare by the labours of the seventeenth century. The University of Cambridge founded a great school of anatomists, which attracted not only students from Oxford, but from beyond the seas.

The work of Caius, the compulsory dissections by students, and the demonstrations by the Regius Professor bore fruit in a brilliant body of writers. Besides Bulleine, Helkiah Crooke, the two Drakes, Sir George Ent, Winston, Briggs, Clopton Havers (the osteologist), Wharton, Croon (the embryologist), Needham, George Joliffe, Martin Lister, Brady, and Edward Tyson (the comparative anatomist), we must especially consider Harvey and Glisson.

9

The immortal Harvey first graduated at Caius College, and then studied at Padua, as Caius himself had done.

Now Fabricius had pointed out the valves of the veins, and Servetus and others had theorized on the circulation, the Galenic teaching on it being that the arterial blood flowed from the heart to the extremities and back by the same vessels, while the venous blood flowed from the liver and back by the veins; but Harvey, by patient observation and experiment, showed clearly that the blood leaves the heart by the arterial system and returns by the venous, while a second circulation also takes blood from the heart to the lungs and brings it back to the heart again. After years of work, he published this exposition in his *Exercitatio Anatomica de Motu Cordis* in 1628. Asellius had discovered the lacteals in 1622, and George Joliffe the lymphatics in 1651, though Bartholini and Radbeck independently pointed them out about the same time.

Francis Glisson, *omnium anatomicorum exactissimus*, as he has been called, became Regius Professor from 1636 to 1677, and wrote his *Anatomy of the Liver* in 1654, and that of the stomach and intestines in 1677. To him we owe the doctrine of irritability, that power of reaction to stimuli which distinguishes living matter from dead; and the discovery that muscles do not increase in bulk when they contract their length ; and also the first clear account of rickets, which he elaborated by discussion at a pathological society, and then published in 1658. At Oxford, also, a Readership of Anatomy was founded in 1624. The Lumleian Lectures date from 1581.

Among other anatomists we should remember Richard Lower, who first performed direct transfusion, and showed that the difference between arterial and venous blood was due to the former having taken up air in the lungs. Mayow went on to prove that it only takes up that part of the air which supports combustion in the tissues in the form of a fermentation, and is essential to every process and change. This came near to an anticipation of oxygen. Thomas Willis held similar views, as he taught that the blood undergoes a slow burning or combustion, kindled by the air in the lungs, and that the processes of the organism are a form of fermentation—*i.e.*, " an internal motion of the particles of a body leading to its perfection or its change into some other form, which we now call metabolism. Fevers and other diseases consist in abnormal fermentation " (Michael Foster, *History of Physiology*). After serving in the Cavalier army, he became Sadlerian Professor in Oxford and then migrated to London, where his discoveries in the nervous system were epoch making. The circle of Willis and his classification of the cranial nerves remain almost unaltered to-day as monuments of his labours. As Richardson says, "anatomy, physiology, chemistry, and the microscope, were now all in a state to be serviceable, and Willis employed them all in his medical studies," though they were, as yet, of less use to the surgeon. The microscope under Malpighi and Leuwenhoek completed the proof of Harvey's doctrine of the circulation by showing the capillaries and the motion of the cells. It did more, for it showed to mankind a new world of objects hitherto invisible and not less important than the terrestrial one which we owe to Columbus.

Cowper, too, and Charlton were discoverers of importance, while Christopher Bennett of Wrington led the way by his post-mortem studies in the pathology of tubercular disease. Edward Tyson's dissections of the chimpanzee, the tapeworm, the embryo shark, and the rattlesnake, laid the foundations of comparative anatomy.

The ordinary medical student was not left in ignorance of these new discoveries. Macalister mentions three eminent men of the Cambridge school who were appointed lecturers on anatomy to the students under the barber surgeon company, and there exists " The manual of the anatomy or dissection of the body of man, containing the enumeration and description of the parts of the same which usually are showed in the public anatomical exercises by Alexander Read, M.D., Fellow of the Physicians' College, and [Foreign] brother of the Worshipful Company of Barber Surgeons. 446 pages, duodecimo. London, 1638."

As a type of the student's handbook of the time this is of special interest. The descriptions show a great advance both in matter and method. The author gives briefly the origin, insertion, and action of each muscle, notices the difference between the contraction and relaxation of a muscle in movements, and the continuance of contraction and relaxation, called "motus tonicus," when the muscle is kept in the same posture.

He says "the brain receives the charge from the soul, the nerve carrieth it to the muscle, and the muscle doth perform the act by the influence of the nerve as the loadstone draweth iron"; but he falls into the old error that the tendinous parts of the muscle are the contractile ones. In describing the circulation, the student is taught that the auricles of the heart receive the blood, and when the heart proper, or ventricles, are dilated they (the auricles) contract, and softly pour in the blood. The right ventricle ministers nourishment to the lungs, but the left communicates the blood to the whole body. In dilatation, blood is drawn in from the vena cava ; in contraction, vital blood is expelled. Between these contrary motions, he adds, we must imagine some rest.   The ventricles are divided by a septum from each other, and no blood can pass through it.

It is clear that the student in the reign of Charles I. was expected to be well up in Harvey's doctrine of the circulation, though the *Exercitatio* was only ten years old.

CHAPTER V

1700 TO 1800 A.D.

1. GENERAL SURVEY OF THE TIMES

THE progress of civilization in Europe during the eighteenth century was at first steady, though marked by fierce wars, but new ideals were springing up, which finally produced great revolutions such as that in France, and altered the whole framework of society.

We are accustomed to think of the period in England as quiet and unromantic, but here, too, it was full of extraordinary political and social changes which are apt to be overlooked. The nation went through seven great wars, of which the shortest lasted seven years. It was the chief period of "the Expansion of England," in which this little insular State in the northern seas became the possessor of a new world in India and America. The social and economic changes were far reaching. The need of food led to the final abolition of the wasteful communal agriculture—the open field system—and to the development of scientific farm-

ing and of stock breeding, which gave to the world
new breeds of cattle and made Britain the stud
farm of the world.   The new use of coal for the
manufacture of iron rendered possible a development of machinery and technical skill in workmen
which revolutionized industry, and produced the
greatest material advance in historical times.   Without this the steam-engine, railroads, and most modern
conquests over nature would have been impossible.
The crystallized socialism and regulation of the
past broke down with the advent of the great
factory system and the doctrines of *laisser faire*.
New towns and new institutions sprang up, and the
population increased rapidly, though unforeseen
hardships affected great masses of the working
classes.   Whilst medicine and surgery shared in the
general advance of science and art, the old organization of education and licensing went to pieces, and
before the end of the century no qualifications were
necessary for practice.   In the revolt against the
restrictions of the old socialism and State regulation individual competition became rampant, and
men preferred the anarchy of unlicensed practice
to an improved form of medical organization, and
they got it.   However, new and fruitful means of
voluntary education were developed both in
England, Scotland, and Ireland, of which large
numbers of students availed themselves to obtain

a thorough knowledge of their art.   The popularity
and success of the new medical schools was so
great that they more than replaced the old system,
both in the number of men they turned out and in
the knowledge and skill of their most distinguished
pupils, but the disappearance of State control over
medical practice and the absence of any public
guarantee of a man's qualifications led to a flood
of charlatans and quacks.   In the seventeenth
century they had been kept in check with difficulty
by the various authorities, but now they flourished
everywhere.   Joanna Stevens, with her cure for
calculi; Chevalier Taylor, the supposed eye surgeon ;
Graham, the purveyor of "celestial beds"; bone-
setters and patent medicine vendors of every kind,
whose exploits form the bulk of most anecdotes of
medicine, grew wealthy by the contributions they
wrung from rich and poor.

2. THE REVIVAL OF HOSPITALS

For two centuries this country had been practically without hospitals for the sick poor or for
the training of students and nurses.   Their revival
was one of the greatest social achievements of the
eighteenth century, the first sign of the humanitarian
and social movement which was to come.

Out of the wreck of the numerous institutions
which had been engulfed, two London houses

first time we find (1) the expenses were met by
voluntary subscriptions; (2) the staff served without fees or salary; and (3) the poor were admitted
without fees, such as barred the way to the older
institutions.   The movement spread in a marvellous
way.   In Edinburgh the Royal College of Physicians
had begun to give gratuitous help to the poor in1682,
and they finally started the Royal Infirmary in 1729.
Aberdeen followed in 1739.   At Winchester, under
Dean Alured Clarke, an infirmary was opened in
1736.   In 1737 Bristol opened another, and before
long the great towns vied with each other in building and supporting a crowd of new hospitals on
the same principles.   Garrison enumerates twenty
in England and six in Scotland.   Thomas Guy had
already munificently founded his great hospital on
the pattern of St. Bartholomew's and St. Thomas's
in 1725.   St. George's Hospital was started by
some members of the Westminster Society in 1734 ;
the London arose in 1740 to meet the needs of
the eastern districts; and the Middlesex in 1745.
Steevens in Dublin left his estates in 1710 to form
a hospital, which was opened in 1733.   The Jervis
Street and Mercer's Hospitals were opened in 1728
and 1734 ; the Cork Hospital as early as 1721.

The Lying-in Hospital in Dublin, 1745, and Queen
Charlotte's in 1764, and hospitals for the insane
were among the first of the specialist institutions.

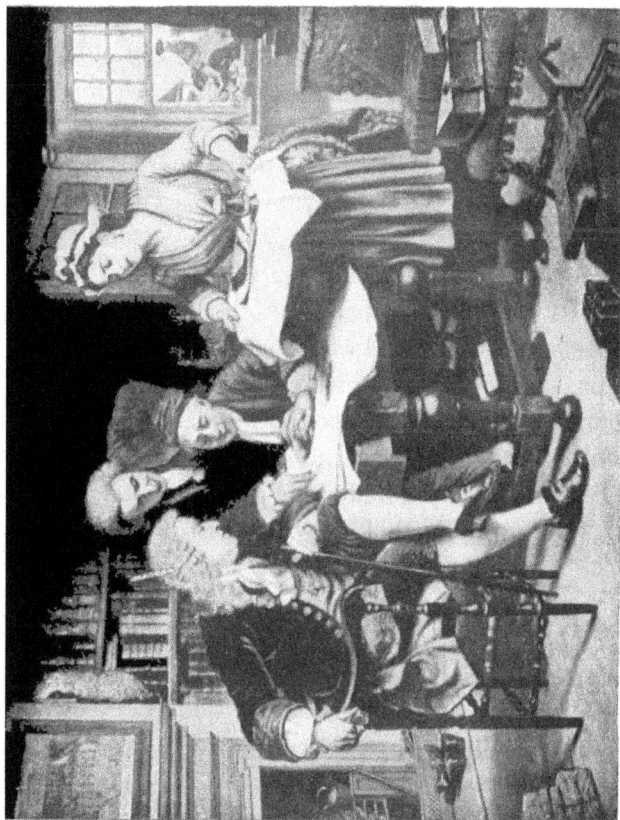

THOMAS GUY, FOUNDER OF GUY'S HOSPITAL,

CONFERRING WITH DR. MEAD, THE PHYSICIAN, AND MR. STEAR, THE ARCHITECT, UPON THE PLAN OF THE BUILDING.

From the original oil-painting by C. W. Cope. R.A., in Guy's Hospital.

The whole movement was extraordinary in its extent and sudden development, and is curiously like the hospital enthusiasm in the twelfth century. It hardly seems to have spread to the Continent with the vigour of the earlier movement, though the Charité in Berlin, 1727, the Allgemeines Krankenhaus in Vienna, 1784, and several French and Russian institutions date from this period.

In one respect the results of the eighteenth century outburst were much greater than those of the twelfth, inasmuch as the new system of medical schools attached to hospitals found its opportunity in the crowd of new institutions.

3. ORGANIZATION OF SURGERY ABROAD AND AT HOME

Surgery on the Continent during this century made little progress.   German and Italian influence and achievements were almost nil, and French surgery, though good, was productive of little but sundry improvements in technique, such as the screw tourniquet of Petit, and Chopart's amputation of the foot.   Frederick the Great found such an absence in Germany of surgeons that he had to engage a body of French surgeons for his troops. Still, a few were trained in Berlin at the new Med.-Chirurgical College (1724) and its hospital, the Charité (1727), from which finally the Kaiser

Wilhelm's Academie has been developed.   Similar colleges were formed in Dresden (1748), Vienna (1785), and Petrograd.

The influence, wealth, and energy of La Peyrouse led to a great advance in France, where Louis XV. created five professorships at St. Côme, abolished the barber surgeons, and raised the status of surgeons. After the foundation of the Academy of Surgery (1731) and the foundation of four professorships at Montpellier, the teaching of surgery in France became the best in the world till it was disorganized by the Revolution.   For a time all the medical and surgical colleges were abolished, and a licence to practise was granted to anyone on paying certain fees.   The resulting anarchy was curiously like that which, as we shall see, obtained in Great Britain at the end of the century.

In Great Britain the barber surgeons were in full power at the beginning of the century, both in London, Dublin, Newcastle, Norwich, Bristol, and York.   The surgeons in the companies got into their hands more and more of the management and of the funds, causing discontent among the non-surgical members, but as long as the legal monopoly of practice continued, these troubles were capable of adjustment.   The law courts, however, began to ignore the act of Elizabeth, 1563, upon which the monopoly of the gilds had come to depend for enforcement (see Privy Council register, October 29, 1669, in G. Unwin's *Industrial Organization in the Sixteenth and Seventeenth Centuries*, p. 252), and their powers became precarious. If the gild could not guarantee the monopoly of practice, there was no use in belonging to it. Various causes influenced public opinion against the old syndicalist system of regulation of trade. There had long been a gradual loosening of the hold of the gilds upon the callings they represented (see again G. Unwin's *Gilds and Companies of London*, pp. 341-351), bitter fights at the time of the Great Rebellion against the monopolies which the Government was driven to create in the absence of sufficient regular taxes, and finally the rise of the economic theory of *laisser faire*, which boldly proclaimed that all action which could be construed as a restraint of trade was against the public utility. Thus the whole of the socialist system of regulation was exchanged for pure individualism, where every man was left to fight for himself, one of the usual cycles of change which recur in human history. No doubt in many trades other causes, such as the rise of the great factory mode of production, helped on the movement, but close corporations were doomed, and with them fell the strange but great companies to which the State and the Law had entrusted the education and licensing of surgeons.

The London Company had long shown signs of the coming division. In 1643 it was agreed that at the election of Wardens all members who belonged to other callings and professions should be reckoned barbers as opposed to the surgeons' group, which was indeed laid down in the charter of Henry VII. In 1684, after many disputes had gone on, the surgeons proposed separation of the company into two bodies, and presented a petition to Parliament which came to nothing. Again, in 1744 they supported a second petition, and the barbers in reply pointed out that at the time of their incorporation, 1540, they were a distinct body within the company, and did not even then practise surgery; that the surgeons had full opportunity of discussing surgical matters alone; and, finally, that the separation which now existed in Edinburgh, Glasgow, and Paris was not a sufficient precedent. However, the House decided against them, and the company was divided into two on May 2, 1745. *A new company of surgeons* was thus formed, taking over the Gale and Arris bequests for lectures, the right of choosing surgeons for the army as well as for the navy, and the old exemption from serving on juries and parish offices. The fees for admission were reduced from £100 to £25, and the company started as the licenser and educator of London surgeons, leaving to the barbers the ancient hall, the paintings, silver, and books which had accumulated for ages.   But the fates were against them, their monopoly had practically gone, and they failed to create themselves the body which should rule and advance surgery.   " Your theatre is without lectures, your library without books," said their Master in 1790.

At last, in 1800, on March 22, a royal charter was obtained for a new body, the Royal College of Surgeons in London, which would not be one of the city companies, but a head and teacher for all surgeons in the realm.   Great as its aims and duties were, it had few or no compulsory powers, and the profession was thrown open to every pretender without check.   The anarchy of unlicensed practice for another half century had full scope.

In Glasgow the barbers put up with the unpleasant position of paying their fees to the faculty, while they had no voice in making regulations. In 1701 they appealed through the union or house of the gilds to the City Council, and prayed for redress of their grievances, or else that they could be separated from the surgeons.   The Council found in their favour, since the surgeons had used the common funds for various purposes, while they excluded the barbers from office.   The same faults were found in 1703.   Finally, in 1719 complete separation took place, the surgeons renounced the letter of deaconry, but remained as a part of the ancient faculty, which ended the attempt of 1656 to graft the usual British system on to Peter Lowe's Faculty of Physicians and Surgeons.

In Bristol violent disputes took place between the two bodies in the company. In 1739 thirty-two members appealed to the City Council against the "other part of the company called surgeons." The Master and Wardens reply against these "uneasie members," and another petition in 1740 prays for a revision of their ordinances. In 1742 the Surgeons' Company, as it was called, appeared for the last time in a civic procession "marching with music" at the opening of the Exchange. Without any fresh legislation the surgeons left the company, and no penalties were enforced, though we find two of the surgeons who were attached to the new infirmary gave courses of anatomy as late as 1746 in the anatomical theatre of the barber surgeons' hall, which was a fine new building. Very soon, however, the hall was turned to other uses, and the students who walked the hospital had to find classes elsewhere.

In Newcastle-on-Tyne the company, which, as in other cities, came under municipal recognition and rule in 1442, built themselves as late as 1730 a new surgeons' hall with beautiful rose gardens around it, and an anatomical theatre. Though no quarrels have come to light, and it seems to have been a vigorous school of surgery, to which students of good social position were attracted, a similar decay fell over it, and we hear nothing of it for a century, till the transfer of the hall and theatre to the Newcastle School of Medicine in 1834. The company still exists as such, though all tradition of surgical teaching has passed away. In York, in Norwich, Salisbury, Chester, and other centres, the companies disappear without disturbance during the eighteenth century, and fade from remembrance.

The Dublin company had fallen on evil days, in spite of a new charter in 1687. A rival society of surgeons appeared about 1721, and the old body became moribund. In its place the Royal College of Surgeons of Ireland was created in 1784. Indeed, long before this Trinity College in 1712 had started a medical school, which has ever since continued to flourish, more especially since its endowment by Sir Patrick Dun in 1744. The companies in Limerick, Cork, and Youghal have left no records of interest.

The Edinburgh company at the end of the seventeenth century was practically in the hands of the surgeons, who seized on the funds and ruled supreme; but the barbers brought an action in 1718 and proved that they were originally on an equality in the corporation, and that the surgeons practising as such had alone to pass examinations in surgery and anatomy. This was undoubtedly the rule in English companies where the two crafts were conjoined. However, the court gave the barbers then existing a fair share of the funds and a right to manage their own affairs. In effect, it finally separated the two bodies. The Corporation of Surgeons had already in 1697 built a new hall, and begun teaching anatomy with vigour. In 1720 they formed other lectureships, and finally created the "extramural school," which has gone on to the present time.

4. The Hospital Schools

Thus the barber surgeons' companies disappeared in the early part of the century, having lost their monopoly of practice in the towns and with it the value of their licences.

The universities and the bishops had also ceased to be of any importance as licensing bodies, with the exception of the new schools at Edinburgh, Dublin, and indeed at Glasgow and Aberdeen. The London Corporation or Company of Surgeons was a failure. Surgical education had lost its old organization, but it now enters on a new career. Two classes of fresh schools arose : first the private schools such as those conducted by Smellie, Cullen, Black, Blizard, and Maclaurin, and the Windmill

Street school under the Hunters, Baillie, and Cruickshank. These did good work in the absence of any great public institutions in England, but they were transient, and, of course, had no licensing powers. Secondly, the endless new hospitals afforded a field for teaching of a fresh type, and in every city a school of medicine and surgery attached to the local hospital or infirmary for the students "walking the hospital" began to grow up. The system of apprenticeship had alone survived from the fourteenth century, and the medical men attached to the new hospitals obtained the privilege of taking their apprentices to assist them with their cases in the wards, and soon made efforts to provide systematic teaching for them and clinical instruction in the wards. The schools, then, grew up as the result of individual enterprise, but the system was found to be of such enormous advantage to the student and to increase the efficiency of the hospitals so greatly that it quickly replaced the old institution.

We have noticed the early beginnings of the movement in St. Bartholomew's, where the growth of the school led to the foundation of a museum of anatomy and surgery under the care of John Freke in 1726, and the institution of anatomical lectures in 1734 under Edward Nourse. Percivall Pott began to lecture in 1765, the Pitcairns lectured on medicine, and John Abernethy from 1787 on surgery, physiology, and anatomy to great crowds of students. At St. Thomas's, where we saw that students existed in 1695, Cheselden, though a lecturer and Master of the barber surgeons, began to give a course on anatomy in 1720. The London Hospital received students in 1742, and took over Blizard's teachers in 1768. Guy's Hospital followed in 1769 with surgical lectures. In the provinces the same thing happened; for instance, in Bristol Messrs. Page and Ford began lectures on anatomy in 1746, and were followed by others, though a complete medical school was not organized before 1828. On the Continent the movement also went on at Vienna, Prague, Pavia, Jena, and at Paris in 1780. Thus in England the apprenticeship system was now supplemented by lectures on anatomy and other subjects at the new hospitals, and clinical instruction in the wards, but no licensing body tested the proficiency of the students, so that by the end of the century the practice of surgery was open to anyone, whatever his qualifications were.

In Scotland the universities began to take such a brilliant part in combining lectures with clinical teaching that they attracted students from all parts of the world, and formed the greatest medical school in the British Isles and perhaps in Europe.

5. The Universities

Edinburgh, for a century after its foundation in
1592, took no share in medical study.   At last, in
1720, the City Council appointed Alexander Monro,
who was lecturing in the hall of the corporation of
surgeons, and made him Professor of Anatomy.
In 1726 they went further, and created four other
professors from his old colleagues, and granted
them power to give degrees.   A Professor of Midwifery was added to the surgeons and physicians.
A hospital was started in 1729, and the foundation
of the Royal Infirmary took place in 1738.   The
students increased in an extraordinary way; nearly
13,000 had studied medicine under the two first
Monros by 1790, and at that date the students in
all faculties rose to about 1,200 under the Principal-
ship of Robertson, the historian.   Here was a
surprising change.   The connection of medical and
surgical studies with university teaching had
almost died out in Britain, and now the most
flourishing school of the time was growing up in
a vigorous and crowded university.   It recalled
the days of the early Italian schools, when classical,
philosophical, and medical studies were carried
on in the same place and with a common enthusiasm.

Students again flocked to the new school not

only from Britain, but from every part of the world, and the union of hospital and university teaching in able hands offered a combination of practical and intellectual training of the highest value.   Ireland, too, followed on similar lines, and at Dublin the new school in Trinity College began to educate a group of able men.   In England the universities were unaffected by the movement, though hospitals were founded in both of them ; but in Berlin, Vienna, Paris, Leyden, and other continental centres, surgery and medicine still found homes in or alongside of flourishing universities.

6. English Surgeons

A few great surgeons, such as Cheselden and Pott, did good work ; but the greatest advance of surgery dates only from the time of John Hunter, when it ceased to be a "mere technical mode of treatment, and began to take its place as a branch of scientific medicine, firmly grounded in physiology and pathology " (Garrison).

William Cheselden (1688-1752), born, like Tennyson, at Somersby in Lincoln, was a pupil of Cowper the anatomist.   He took the Grand Diploma of the barber surgeons in 1710, and became lecturer on anatomy in 1711.   In 1719 he was elected a surgeon at St. Thomas's, and later on at St. George's

Hospital. He was Junior Warden of the barber surgeons in 1744, and after the disruption was Master of the new company of surgeons, 1746. The lateral lithotomy which he perfected in 1727 has remained almost unaltered ever since. He had fame, too, as an ophthalmic surgeon, and his artistic skill may be seen in some of the plates which he drew for his great *Atlas of the Human Bones, or Osteographia.* His marvellous rapidity in operating is shown by his doing a lithotomy in fifty-four seconds (Garrison), a matter of importance when the patient had no anæsthetic. A friend of Pope and Hans Sloane, he attained great popularity both in and outside of his professional work.

William Shippen (1736-1788), an American trained at Edinburgh, was the first Professor of Surgery and Anatomy in the medical department of Pennsylvania, and was made Surgeon-General of the United States army. Besides his work in teaching obstetrics, his success in organizing the army medical service, after the efforts of J. Morgan and Church, are his chief claims to remembrance.

Percivall Pott (1714-1788) took the Grand Diploma of the barber surgeons in 1736, and was made assistant surgeon at St. Bartholomew's, 1744, where his lectures became crowded with students. His description of the fracture of the fibula with

dislocation, which bears his name, is due to his
fall from his horse at Westminster, and the injury
he then incurred. The account he gives of this
injury is as follows:

" When the fibula breaks within two or three
inches of its lower extremity, the inferior fractured
end falls inwards towards the tibia, that extremity
of the bone which forms the outer ankle is turned
somewhat outward and upward, and the tibia
having lost its proper support is forced off from
the astragalus inwards, by which means the weak
bursal or common ligament of the joint is violently
stretched if not torn, and the strong ones which
fasten the tibia to the astragalus and os calcis are
always lacerated, thus producing a perfect fracture
and a partial dislocation to which is sometimes
added a wound in the integuments. . . . All the
tendons which pass behind or under, or are attached
to the extremities of the tibia and fibula or os calcis,
have their natural direction so altered that they all
contribute to the distortion of the foot and that by
turning it outward and upward. . . .

" It is extremely troublesome to put to rights,
still more so to keep it in order, and unless managed
with address and skill is very frequently productive
of lameness and deformity ever after. . . . But if
the position of the limb be changed, if by laying it
on its outside with the knee moderately bent, the
muscles forming the calf of the leg and those which
pass behind the fibula and under the os calcis are
all put in a state of relaxation and non-resistance,
all this difficulty and trouble do in general vanish
immediately, the foot may easily be placed right,

the joint reduced, and by maintaining the same disposition of the limb everything will in general succeed very happily. Two kinds of fracture there are, and only two, that I can recollect relative to the limbs which do not admit of the bent position of the joints, I mean that of the processus olecranon at the elbow and that of the patella. In these a straight position of the arm and leg is necessary."
—*Remarks on Fractures and Dislocations.*

Besides this, he is famous for the spinal disease due to caries, which he first explained, and for his writings on head injuries, hernia, and dislocations.

Sir John Pringle (1707-1782) was Surgeon-General of the British armies from 1742 to 1758, and obtained the neutralization of military hospitals in war which became part of the Geneva Convention. He laid the foundation of modern military sanitation, fought for better ventilation, and wrote a monumental work on the diseases of the army.

John Hunter (1728-1793) left behind him a reputation which far outpasses that of any of his contemporaries. His passionate love of science and extraordinary capacity for work are the keystone of his life. As a lad he was indeed inactive and aimless, like Darwin, but he went to London, and under the help and guidance of his elder brother William he found his deepest interest in anatomy, and quickly became a teacher. Then he became a pupil of Cheselden and Pott, and

finally a surgeon at St. George's Hospital. He
gained experience of gunshot wounds in the
expedition to Belle Isle, 1761, and in a Spanish
campaign, and was finally made Surgeon-General.
As a teacher and as a brilliant surgeon he was
unrivalled. At St. George's, where students
crowded after him, he urged that a real teaching
school should be organized. He was the first great
pathologist, and collected in his private museum
some 13,000 specimens. His studies on inflamma-
tion, the repair of tendons, phlebitis, the hard
chancre, and numerous other subjects, are the foundation of our present knowledge in those matters.
His operation for aneurism due to arterial disease
was not absolutely novel, but he first showed its
value by arguments gleaned from anatomy, physiology, animal experiment, post-mortem findings, and
other fields. He built up an immense practice, but
continued his scientific researches, collections, and
dissections, with the extraordinary industry which
was peculiar to him. He brought into the study of
surgery the habit of testing everything by experiment and observation instead of relying upon
theories. He taught men to look on surgery as
a branch of natural science which must be studied
in relation to other branches. As Stephen Paget
expresses his aim : Comparative anatomy must be
made to explain human. Pathology and physiology

both of men and animals must be made to throw
every light on anatomy and surgery. "Don't
think ; try," wrote Hunter—that is, don't waste
time in theorizing on doubtful and scanty facts, but
collect all the facts possible, test and collate them.
He collected every animal, plant, or fossil, which
could be of scientific interest. His leisure hours
were filled up with observations on such subjects
as hibernation, healing of wounds, the development
of an egg, and the habits of animals. Even his
own illness produced twenty quarto pages of notes
on the symptoms. For he reasoned that the
pathology of angina pectoris was unknown, and
every scrap of knowledge based on observation
should be preserved. Papers before the Royal
Society on animal physiology, the formation of his
great museum, his correspondence with scientific
men and explorers, the care and observation of his
collection of living animals, were only part of his
unwearied labours. It is not too much to say
that the difference between the surgical thought of
to-day and that of the eighteenth century is chiefly
due to the growth of that scientific method and
spirit which was Hunter's great characteristic.

His death was as hurried as his life. Frequent
paroxysms of angina had attacked him from time
to time, when one day he drove to St. George's to
speak at a committee. He became excited by the

opposition he met with at the board.   An attack came on, he left the room, went a few steps, groaned, and died then and there.

John Abernethy (1764-1831) a devoted pupil of Hunter's, and himself a teacher of great power, was made assistant surgeon at St. Bartholomew's in 1787.   Here his lectures were a great success, and attracted crowds of hearers.   An operation which he did has been cited as one of the earliest in nerve surgery.   He divided a nerve in the arm for violent and continued pain, and was able to show that after the removal of half an inch reunion took place and sensibility in time returned (J. S. Billings).   He was also the first to tie the external iliac artery, and in 1789 ligatured the common carotid.

7. ANATOMY

Anatomy made great strides at Paris, Edinburgh, Copenhagen, and Berlin, as well as in London, though the advance of the science was less rapid than in the seventeenth century.

Cowper's treatise on the urethral glands, Cheselden's work on the bones, and Smellie and Douglas's discoveries were followed in England by the epoch-making researches of the Hunters.   William Hunter built the great anatomical theatre and museum in Great Windmill Street, and wrote the history of anatomy.   His atlas of the pregnant uterus, his discovery of the separate fœtal circulation and the decidua reflexa, are only a few of his contributions to the science.

In Edinburgh the three Monros held the chair of anatomy in succession for 126 years, and raised that city to the first rank as an effective school.

Pitcairn, says Hingston Fox, had tried for years after his return from Leyden to get the city to set up a medical school. At last they appointed Alexander Monro as teacher of anatomy. He had been brought up by his father from boyhood to take this very position. He had learned anatomy of Cheselden and Douglas in London. At Leyden he studied under Albinus, and was a favourite pupil of Boerhaave. His father's efforts collected fifty-seven students to hear his first course of lectures, which he delivered in the old Surgeons' Hall in 1720, when he was only twenty-two years of age. He made his mark at the outset as a teacher, and for thirty-eight years he lectured to an ever-increasing class. His son followed him as professor, and his grandson succeeded in due time. Professorships of anatomy were established or revived in all the British universities, but at Oxford and Cambridge there was none of the success and enthusiasm which marked the earlier movement under Caius and Glisson. Stephen Hales, an English country clergyman, investigated the blood-pressure, and William Hewson the coagulation of the blood, and both of them did work which still remains of value. The advance of physiology, and even of chemistry, began to make anatomy more fruitful. In Berne and Göttingen, Von Haller was by far the greatest physiologist of the day, the founder of recent physiology, as Garrison calls him, a man whose extraordinary energy reminds us of Hunter.

Réaumur and Spallanzani threw light on the nature and action of gastric juice, while another group of scientists—Black, Priestley, Lavoisier, and others—finally explained the riddle of respiration.

CHAPTER VI

1800 TO 1850 A.D.

1. GENERAL SURVEY OF THE TIME

THE first half of the nineteenth century was marked by a new Renaissance, the latest revival, as Dr. Payne has pointed out, of the Greek spirit and method of the experimental investigation of nature. We are reminded in it of the phenomena of the twelfth and sixteenth centuries, when a similar Renaissance had taken place and like progress was made. We can already perceive that this period has not been the least fruitful of the various revivals.

In England especially it was an age of wonders mixed with the drabbest respectability. After our long struggle in the Napoleonic wars, when we withstood the whole force of Europe, England emerged stronger than ever, with a world-wide empire, a mastery of the seas so complete that we could hand back without fear to our neighbours their colonies, the whole of which had fallen into our hands.

Then followed forty years of peace, when the revival of science had time to develop and the material results began to appear. These were so great as to form the strongest incentive to further efforts, even if the disinterested love of knowledge were absent, but, in fact, a real enthusiasm for science had grown up. The appearance of the first steamboat, the first railway train, the first telegraph, and the first practical compound microscope mark the arrival of a new age, and these gains were rivalled in other fields of work by the discoveries of the mathematicians, the chemists and the astronomers. In history a new method sprang up from the date of Gibbon's work, and the bounds of its subject-matter were enlarged by the discoveries of Egyptian and Assyrian life, of Sanscrit, and prehistoric lore.

In every direction new ideals and hopes came to the front, and, as in earlier revivals, the outburst of a school of romantic poets, such as Shelley, Byron, Scott, and Wordsworth, marked the fresh spirit of the time.

A humanitarian movement echoing the broken ideals of Rousseau and the dreams of the European Revolution found vent in the emancipation of slaves, in the Factory Acts, in the Poor Law and political reforms, and in determined efforts to make sanitary science a real protector of the poor.

Population doubled and trebled in a brief period, leading to great food difficulties and various changes in the Corn Laws.

The individualism and competition which ruled at the beginning of the period had their advantages in stimulating research, but their disadvantages began to be felt, and once more combinations and societies in every calling, profession, trade, or study arose, and even in some cases State regulation.

The Great Exhibition of 1851 summed up the popular enthusiasm for science, and for the new and fruitful arts, as well as the belief that wars had come to an end.

In this seething new life surgery and medicine acquired higher ideals, and during the period began to obtain such great help from the allied sciences that at the end of it they were in a position to make the enormous strides which characterize the modern period. This last, however, falls outside the scope of this volume.

2. The Position of Surgery at Home and Abroad

J. S. Billings, while remarking that more progress has been made since 1800 than in the preceding two thousand years, sums up the position of surgery in 1800 by saying that the surgeon had little more knowledge than had Hippocrates of the chief causes of danger after operations, such as suppuration, pyæmia, or tetanus, and groped wildly for means to avoid them.

He had no clinical thermometer, and could only guess at temperature and fever; no hypodermic syringe, no anæsthetics, no definite knowledge of the importance of blood saving, or of the best means of doing it. He knew nothing of plastic surgery, of tenotomy, of the ophthalmoscope, or of the use of the microscope in diagnosis, and had merely learned how to ligature arteries and to treat ordinary wounds in a simple, sensible way. The really great surgeon of that day, who was bold, cool, and skilful, could perform most of the great operations, but such men were few and far between.

In the first half of the century—*i.e.*, before the scientific discoveries made possible the great advances of the modern period—surgery undoubtedly gained many solid victories, and this was largely due to the combination of the study of anatomy and pathology with surgery, a fashion which Hunter created, and which we see exemplified in all the best surgeons of the time. Men like Astley Cooper, Brodie, Bell, and Liston were not content with attaining unrivalled dexterity and swiftness in operating, but they laboured incessantly in dissections, in the collection and study of specimens of diseased organs, and in physiology. In spite of their limitations due to the absence of anæsthetics and antiseptics, they devised endless improvements in the recognized operations, which their wider knowledge dictated; as well as new fields of work. Thus we find growing up conservative surgery under Fergusson and Syme, with its preference for resections and excision of joints in place of amputations; a new ophthalmic surgery under Bowman and others; lithotomy and lithotrity of an improved type under Key, Liston, and Crosse of Norwich; attempts at ovariotomy by Lizars, Morgan, Clay, and later on by Spencer Wells. This was also being developed in America under McDowell, an Edinburgh student, and the Attlees. Even laryngology was advancing under Liston and Babington before Garcia's invention of the laryngoscope in 1855, and we must not forget the efforts of Astley Cooper and others to place the treatment of hernia and malignant growths on a sound basis.

The first steps in the development of anæsthetics, too, come into this period. Various narcotics had been used from early times. They are described by Theodoric and Chauliac, and, indeed, by the ancients. Hypnotism was employed by Elliotson in 1843, and by J. Esdaile for one hundred operations in India in 1845. About 1800 nitrous oxide

was the subject of endless experiments by Humphry
Davy, working in Dr. Beddoe's Pneumatic Institute
at Bristol, and was actually employed by Wells
for dental operations in 1844. Ether had been
tried apparently by Crawford W. Long in 1839,
and at last Morton, also an American, made it a
success between 1844 and 1846. It was at once
taken up by Robert Liston, by Syme, by Pirogoff,
and Sir James Simpson. The latter, however, exchanged it for chloroform in 1847, which became,
especially in Edinburgh, the favourite anæsthetic.

In France, in spite of the disorganization of the
medical schools in the early days of the Revolution,
a group of brilliant surgeons appeared. Some of
them were of the military class, such as Larrey,
of whom Napoleon said in his will that he was
"the most virtuous man I have ever known." He
wrote copiously, though serving for twenty-two
years in various campaigns, where he was present
at over four hundred engagements. He also
devised endless measures for the benefit of the
soldiers, amongst others the *ambulances volantes.*
His colleague, Percy, first organized a corps of
litter bearers or field ambulances in Italy.

Dupuytren was the greatest surgeon and teacher
of the time, and the founder of pathological studies
in France. He is remembered for his skill in
fractures, subcutaneous operations, and his great

museum lectures, which attracted students from all parts of the world. Lisfranc, the deviser of many new operations ; Delpech, the orthopædist ; Nélaton, the pathologist, and inventor of the probe named after him ; Malgaine, a skilled operator and anatomist, who became the greatest historian of medicine ; and Broca, the brain surgeon, and founder of modern anthropology, are only a few of the men who maintained the high rank of French surgery.

Germany was not specially distinguished in the early part of the century, but Von Graefe revived plastic surgery, and was followed in this and in the professorship at Berlin by Dieffenbach, a really able surgeon. Military surgery was greatly advanced by Stromeyer, and the younger Von Langenbeck. Pirogoff, the Russian, too, was a brilliant military surgeon and teacher, and a great anatomist, who introduced the method of study by sections of frozen bodies.

On the whole the period was marked by many men of talent and of extraordinary energy and devotion. In America, too, much good surgery was done, especially by V. Mott and the younger Warren, both pupils of Astley Cooper.

In these pre-Listerian days one battle against sepsis must be mentioned. Scmmelweiss, the Hungarian, was in 1846 horrified at the mortality from puerperal fever in the Vienna hospital, and found that students came direct from the dissecting room to one puerperal ward where the death rate was highest. At the death of a colleague from a dissection wound he noted that the post-mortem appearances were the same as in the women who died of puerperal fever (Garrison's *History*, p. 370). He took precautions at once to alter the customs, and made the assistants disinfect their hands, with the result that the mortality fell from 10 per cent. to a little over 1 per cent. Henceforward he proclaimed the infectious nature of the disease. Wendell Holmes had already written in the same direction, but fierce opposition was stirred up against them both, and the acceptance of their teaching was delayed for many years.

One difficulty experienced by the surgeons of the time, due largely to want of organization, was the crude and undeveloped position of nursing. Illeducated, untrained, and undisciplined, the nurses of the period as a rule were unreliable, and without any idea of the possibilities of their art. In the British Army the state of things was even worse. There were no trained dressers or nurses, no ambulances or special organization for carrying off the wounded. The surgeon himself, before the Royal Warrant of 1858 which followed the Crimean fiascos, had no power even to recommend to the commanding officer measures for the protection of the men's health. There were found brilliant surgeons in the Napoleonic wars, and later ; but for the generality of army surgeons there were no means for study or incentives to undertake it, and no organization for the care of the sick. The result was the hideous medical failure in the Crimea.

3. The Chief British Surgeons

Sir Astley Paston Cooper, 1768-1841, was a pupil of Cline, and for a short time of his uncle, William Cooper, but more than all he was influenced by the teaching of John Hunter. He became the chief of those disciples of Hunter who made his scientific ideas predominant in this country. He was possessed of much of Hunter's restless energy and his devoted passion for anatomy. Hunter was a rough prophet, and as a lecturer he was hardly intelligible. Cooper in this respect was a complete contrast. Brought up in good society, he was a genial, kindly, vivacious man, very handsome, and usually dressed in blue with white breeches, his hair fastened in a queue. He had a real gift both for speaking and for teaching the hundred or more students who crowded into his wards. He had fathomed the scientific aims of Hunter, and his great object was to get men to take a deeper view of the problems of surgery. He changed his lectures into demonstrations so as to interest his students in the principles he laid down. " Read the book of Nature" was his favourite saying—*i.e.*, by observation and experiment find out what the real facts are. For a short time he had studied in Edinburgh, where he gained the esteem of the gruff Gregory and others; then he studied under Desault in Paris, but was obliged to flee for his life with his young bride during the Reign of Terror in the Revolution.

He was appointed surgeon at Guy's in 1800, and threw himself indefatigably into his hospital work, into his teaching, and dissecting. Experimental investigations on animals preceded his great feats of ligaturing the common carotid, the external iliac, and the abdominal aorta. He was made Professor of Comparative Anatomy at the Hunterian Museum, and commenced researches on hernia, which he published in 1804. Meanwhile he acquired the best practice in London, attending the Prime Minister and many of the nobility. Suddenly, with hardly any warning, he was called on to remove a large sebaceous cyst from the head of the King himself. He dissected it out with the few instruments at hand, but he knew the likelihood of erysipelas following and the professional ruin which awaited him if it went wrong. A miserable

week it was for him, but the King recovered,
created him a baronet, and remained a constant
friend. To the poorest of his patients in his clinics
Cooper showed the same courteous, kindly manner
as he did to his noble patrons. He found time for
investigations on aural surgery, which received the
medal of the Royal Society, and published elaborate
works on injuries of the joints, and diseases of the
testes, and the anatomy of the breast. Occasionally he took a brief holiday at his country farm,
but even there he would carry on his experiments
and dissections at odd moments. At home he
laboured and taught from six in the morning till
after midnight—a wonderful combination of ability
and industry, courtesy and decision.

Sir Benjamin Collins Brodie, 1783-1862, was
another disciple of Hunter's, and, like him, was
attached to the staff of St. George's. He coupled
his anatomical studies, in which he taught for
a time at Great Windmill Street, with physio-
logical research on the influence of the nerves on
the heart and secretion of gastric juice. He wrote
a masterly treatise on the pathology and diseases of
the joints, and another on diseases of the urinary
organs. A brilliant operator and profound
anatomist, he largely developed the new subcutaneous surgery. Like Cooper, he showed
infinite courtesy and kindness equally to poor and

rich, and as he rose to be the recognized leader of his profession he made fewer enemies than any other man. With an income of £10,000 a year, he was mindful of the needs of poor patients and students, and at the same time became the friend and adviser of the chief men of the day. The scientific side of surgery remained to the last his chief interest, as it had been that of Hunter, and he was ever seeking from pathology and physiology how disease could be healed.

Robert Liston, 1794-1847, an Edinburgh man, came to London, where he was first attached to the North London Hospital, and then became Professor of Clinical Surgery at the new London University, 1834. In him we find another devoted anatomist, and perhaps the most skilful operator of the age. It is related of him that he would amputate the thigh with only one assistant to hold the leg and tie the ligatures. He himself compressed the artery with his left hand, as he used no tourniquet, and with his right he did all the cutting and sawing. His fame rested largely on his modification of the flap operation, as well as on his removal of the upper jaw and on his improvements in lithotomy and lithotrity.

Sir William Fergusson, 1808-1877, a pupil of Robert Knox, also taught first in Edinburgh, and then came to London in 1840 as Professor at

King's College, and became in turn the foremost operator in London. The development of conservative surgery was the object of much of his labour, by which amputations have been so largely diminished. His operations on cleft palate, excision of joints, and lithotomy are justly famous, and his swiftness in them was so great that it was said of him, " If you only wink you miss the operation altogether."

James Syme, 1799-1870, was appointed to the Royal Infirmary at Edinburgh in 1833, and acquired a huge practice. He had begun life as a teacher of anatomy, and later on did more than perhaps anyone else to substitute excisions for amputations. His writings included *The Principles of Surgery* in 1822, and *Contributions to the Pathology and Practice of Surgery*, 1847, in which the first cases of his amputation at the ankle were described. He appears to have been a genial, cheerful man, ready to welcome any useful discovery such as anæsthetics, which he was one of the first to use.

G. T. Guthrie, 1785-1856, a great military surgeon, accompanied Wellington in the Peninsula and served in North America, and again at Waterloo, where he amputated the leg of a Frenchman at the hip-joint. His treatise on gunshot wounds requiring amputation was the standard treatise on the subject.   It was published in 1815, and he survived to make additions in 1855 during the Crimean War. He was also famed as an ophthalmic surgeon.

Abraham Colles, 1773-1843, studied at Edinburgh, and then became Professor of Surgery in Dublin for thirty-two years, and the chief Irish surgeon of the time. His name is now chiefly remembered for the fracture which he described in 1814, and for the law he enunciated as to the degree of immunity possessed by the healthy mother of a syphilitic child.

Sir Charles Bell will be mentioned later on. His brother John Bell, Key, Travers, Blizard, Wardrop, Hey of Leeds, and Sir William Laurence are among the other great surgeons of the period.

4. The Organization of Surgery

The Royal College of Surgeons in London got their new charter in 1800, and settled in a house in Lincoln's Inn Fields under the rule of a Court of Assistants of twenty-one members, one of whom was to be styled the Master. This was changed by a charter of 1822, which created a President, two Vice-Presidents, and a Council. In 1843 the title was given to it of the Royal College of Surgeons of England, and the Fellowship was created. The Fellows were to have the right of electing the Council, which was now increased to twenty-four. The Court of Examiners for the membership was to be chosen from the Fellows, who in 1844 formed a body of over five hundred persons. The college was made the custodian of Hunter's Museum, which parliament had purchased for £15,000. It was opened in 1813, and was rapidly increased. Small grants were made towards a library, which culminated in the purchase, about 1828, of more than £5,000 worth of books.

The college thus became a licensing body in surgery, and gradually took up educational duties; but its licence was optional, and it was still open to anyone to practise without restriction. Quarrels arose as to the schools which should be recognized as preparing candidates for examination, and by degrees a fair standard was reached.

A great number of general practitioners were apprenticed under the Society of Apothecaries, whose separate charter dated from 1617, and who had materially aided the progress of botany and pharmacology by their laboratories and physic gardens. The apothecaries were supposed to charge only for their drugs, and after they became general medical attendants could not take fees, except when they supplied medicines. This helped on the custom of the endless drugging, which still forms the ideal of the poorer classes. At first every dose was put into a separate bottle with a label tied round the neck, and charged for separately. If a surgeon was called in to operate, however often the apothecary had to attend afterwards or to dress the wound, he could get no fee unless he induced the patient to receive potions and dressings each time ; but even these poorly qualified men were better than the numerous class who had no training at all, or boasted of a purchased diploma from some sham college.

At last the apothecaries in 1815 obtained an Act of Parliament enabling them to hold an examination for all England, and not for Londoners alone, and to prosecute unqualified apothecaries, but for a long time the diploma was strictly limited. For instance, the society could not examine in midwifery, though they took care to compel their students to study it. This was the first statute which reimposed penalties on unlicensed practitioners, and nothing more was done until the great Act of 1858, which allows no practitioner to recover fees, hold public appointments, or sign certificates, unless he has been properly examined and placed on an official register. Even this would have been evaded, but as death registration had been made compulsory, ability to sign these certificates became necessary for practice.

Meanwhile the universities in England had almost given up all teaching of surgery or licensing of practitioners. In Scotland and Ireland the universities and the Royal Colleges both taught and licensed all who chose to take out their diplomas.

We have already seen that, before the gilds and companies disappeared, private learned societies began to be formed, where papers were discussed (instead of at the Tuesday meeting in the company's hall) and where discoveries were announced. In the eighteenth century these multiplied, and in the present period the process went on more rapidly still. Dr. Lettsom had persuaded his friends to form the Medical Society of London in 1773 for thirty physicians, thirty surgeons, and thirty apothecaries, which, though not the first of these bodies, has survived to be the oldest of them now existing. After various vicissitudes, it was amalgamated with the Westminster Society. This latter body had started with the Windmill Street School, and about 1824 numbered a thousand members (J. B. Bailey, *Medical Institutions of London*).

Owing to the dissensions in the Medical Society a new body was formed in 1805, the Royal Medical and Chirurgical Society, which owed much to the exertions of Sir Astley Cooper, its first treasurer, and has since had an uninterrupted career of success up to the present day.

Sir William Blizard and his friends around the

12

London Hospital formed the Hunterian Society in 1818, which is still distinguished by the annual oration. Among the numerous other societies of the time we must not forget the Pathological, founded in 1846, and the Harveian, originally the Western London, in 1831. A similar growth took place in the provinces, which were soon covered by a network of societies, but our space does not permit their enumeration, though we must mention the foundation of the British Medical Association in 1832.

In Scotland three societies date from the eighteenth century: the Edinburgh Harveian (1782), and the Aberdeen Med.-Chirurgical (1789), and the Royal Medical (1737) at Edinburgh. This last owed its origin, curiously enough, to the friendship of six students, who dissected together and then continued to meet informally for discussion. As they qualified, the meetings gradually developed into a society. This in turn became possessed of a house and endowment, and finally of royal patronage. The Edinburgh Med.-Chirurgical (1821), and the Glasgow one of the same name (1814), with the Southern (1844), and Obstetrical (1840), are the chief ones of this period.

This habit of meeting for scientific discussion led to opportunities for debates on professional difficulties and ethics. In former times the gilds and companies had endeavoured to enforce a good moral standard in professional conduct. John of Arderne, Gale, and others, had written against the offenders. Under the eighteenth century individualism, all checks except those of the Royal College of Physicians had disappeared. The standard of professional morality tended to fall to that of the ordinary competitive trader, but with the growth of these new societies it was gradually felt that the confidential status of the medical adviser demanded something higher. As I have said elsewhere (*Edin. Med. Journ.*, Oct., 1918), it was seen that the man who advised useless operations and profited by secret nostrums and lying advertisements was a danger, not only to the public, but also to the more honest practitioner, " who was ready to supply disinterested counsel and service to patients for a direct and definite compensation, apart from expectation of other business gain " (as the *New Statesman* phrases it). Many of the societies formed ethical committees, which settled disputes and ejected members guilty of serious offences. The result has been a most remarkable rise of the ethical standard and behaviour of the practitioner, which was aided by the formation of the General Medical Council with the revival of penal powers under the Act of 1858. That this has not been the least gain of the

century is evident to every reader of novelists of
the Georgian period.

5. The Universities and Medical Schools

The ordinary English student about 1800 was
apprenticed for seven years to some surgeon or
general practitioner, and usually arranged to
" walk a hospital," or to attend a private school of
anatomy, surgery, or medicine, and then tried for a
diploma such as the M.R.C.S. The private schools
were important for a time, but passed away as the
hospital schools became better organized. The
Great Windmill Street School was connected with
Hunter and his followers. It had begun under
Sharp, but was taken over by William Hunter
in 1746, and then existed in Covent Garden.
John Hunter lectured here for a time, and then
Hewson and Cruickshank. After William Hunter's
death in 1783 his nephew, Matthew Baillie, took
it over. A complete course of medicine and
surgery, as well as anatomy, was arranged about
1800, Brodie and Wilson being two of the teachers.
Sir Charles Bell followed about 1812, but the
foundation of University College in 1828 led to the
disappearance of this school, where so many of the
best surgeons had been trained for nearly a
century. The *Webb Street School*, started by
Grainger of Birmingham in 1819, had five years

later some 300 students. It took not only anatomy,
but chemistry, surgery, midwifery, and medicine.
It lasted till 1842, when the reforms at St.
Thomas's led to its absorption. *Dermott's School*
also offered a complete course.   It began in 1833,
and claimed at one time 300 students.   There were
also two purely anatomical schools. *Carpue's in
Dean Street, Soho,* existed from 1800 to 1830.
Carpue was a very able teacher, and extremely
popular.   He had a habit of making each student
in turn demonstrate the same part, so that the
points were repeated till everyone knew them.
Brooke's School in Blenheim Street had 150 students
at its best.   He was regarded as the finest teacher
in London, and was made a F.R.S. for his
researches on the preservation of bodies, which he
injected with saltpetre.   Another hobby of his
was the formation of a museum of comparative
osteology (J. B. Bailey).

The hospital schools in London grew rapidly.
We can only give here the briefest account of them.
St. Bartholomew's continued to attract crowds of
students under Abernethy, Stanley, and Laurence.
St. Thomas's was for a time joined with Guy's for
teaching purposes as the United Hospitals, but this
arrangement came to an end in 1824-1836.   The
London Hospital, where students were taken from
1741 and lectures had begun in 1749, soon gave a

complete course.   In 1783 a block of buildings was opened for the school, largely through the exertions and liberality of Sir W. Blizard, the surgeon.   John Hunter tried in vain to get a complete school at St. George's, but it was at last started in 1831.   Up to then the students had to go for anatomy and other subjects to the Great Windmill Street School. Charing Cross opened its school in 1835, Westminster in 1841, King's College Hospital, 1839.   At Middlesex from 1796 to 1835 there was the same difficulty as at St. George's.   University College Hospital opened in 1828, but its school may be said to date from 1834.

In the provinces, too, there was a rapid growth both of the hospitals where clinical instruction was given and also of complete medical schools.   Thus *Liverpool* boasted two schools of anatomy in 1825, and in 1834 a complete school was formed at the Royal Institute, which ten years later was annexed to the infirmary.   In *Birmingham* Dr. Sands Cox, who had been a student under Astley Cooper and under his friend Grainger at Webb Street, as well as under Dupuytren in Paris, started a movement to found a school, which opened in Temple Row in 1828.   Finally, laboratories and lecture rooms were built in Paradise Street.   The Rev. Dr. Warneford gave it £27,000, and King William a charter.   The Queen's Hospital was founded for clinical teaching, and Queen's College was built as a residence for medical and other students. In *Bristol* various schools of anatomy in the eighteenth century were followed by one in College Green, which taught also chemistry and medicine, in 1828. This became a complete school in 1833. Its prospectus stated that it gave all lectures required by the Apothecaries' Society, and all except six months' work demanded by the College of Surgeons. At *Manchester* the school was established about the same time, though the lectures on surgery and anatomy there had been recognized by the college as early as 1821. *Leeds* also dates from 1832 ; *Sheffield* from 1828, when two private anatomy schools were absorbed.

Thus in England surgical education grew up in special schools apart from universities, with little or no recognition from the State, while, on the other hand, in Scotland and Ireland the five old universities took a leading part, and the schools formed in them at an earlier period continued to flourish. The contrast was remarkable, and both systems had their advocates. Apprenticeship still existed everywhere, but was becoming less frequent. In Scotland we find also other teaching bodies—the Royal Colleges in Edinburgh, the Royal Faculty in Glasgow, with Anderson's and St. Mungo's Colleges. In Ireland, besides Trinity College,

Dublin, there were the Royal College of Surgeons, the Carmichael and Ledwich Schools, and many private schools, such as Crampton's, the Park Street School, and Kirby's. The opening of the Queen's Colleges in 1849 helped some of the provincial schools. Thus at Belfast Dr. McDonnell began giving lectures to the hospital students in 1827, and the Academical Institute had formed a complete school in 1827, which numbered nearly seventy men when it was absorbed by Queen's College.

The Resurrectionists.—Ever since the sixteenth century the supply of bodies for anatomy had caused difficulties. The grant of executed criminals to the London, Edinburgh, and Salisbury companies, and to the Universities of Aberdeen, Cambridge, Edinburgh, and Dublin, had caused riotous outbreaks at times. The London regulations show the extreme care taken to make the most of the subjects, especially as few preservatives were used, and much irregular seizure of bodies took place. In 1750 we read of a suicide who had been buried at the cross-roads near Bristol. A well-known Bristol surgeon dug up the body at night and conveyed it into the city on a pack-horse. In passing the city gate, the body was dragged off and fell to the ground, to the horror of the watchman. However, it was taken to the surgeon's house and laid on a table till morning. The screams of a maid who saw it roused the neighbours, and matters grew so threatening that it was secretly taken back and reburied, only to be dug up again by a fierce mob, who wished to verify and then avenge the rumoured theft of their comrade. When the new medical schools arose, a huge increase of dissections took place, especially as the Hunters and their pupils set the fashion of perpetually dissecting the bodies of men and animals. John Hunter and Astley Cooper spent large sums in buying the carcasses of rare animals, and an amusing tale is told of Cooper purchasing an elephant which had died in the Tower, and having it conveyed to his house in the City. A crowd gathered in the street to see it delivered. It was at last dragged into the coach-yard, but all efforts to get it into the building were fruitless. A screen was hastily erected to form a little check to the curiosity of the excited crowd, and Cooper, with some of his students, set to work in the open air to gradually dissect the beast. It is presumed that he did not wear his usual white silk stockings and breeches during this tedious operation.

With the exception of two or three of the old grants to the universities there was no legal source whence human bodies could be obtained. An Act of 1752 indeed granted the bodies of actual

murderers to surgeons, and at times the bodies
of unclaimed persons dying in hospital were dissected.   Here and there, as at St. Peter's Hospital,
Bristol, the surgeons claimed this as a customary
right, but the demand was so urgent that a
trade grew up with numbers of ruffians, who dug
up recently interred bodies from secluded burial
grounds and sold them to the anatomists.   Even
surgeons and students began to dig for themselves.
The knowledge and dread of this spread through
the country, and people commenced to have
watchers and to fence in their graves with massive
iron cages, such as may still be seen in some old
churchyards.   The high prices paid for bodies led to
more skilful and rapid methods.   Bransby Cooper,
who has given us the lives and adventures of many
of these ruffians, tells us of one man delivering
in a day a dozen bodies, for which he received £12
each.   The trade became as exciting as smuggling,
and evoked as little reprobation; even the magistrates shut their eyes to it when possible, though
individual body-stealers were sometimes imprisoned.
As the medical schools and students increased
rapidly from 1800 to 1830, the demand for bodies
and the public irritation increased equally.   At
Cambridge a savage mob sacked the anatomical
school and museum on the reports of a body
having been stolen.   I well remember an old friend,

many years after, whom I was showing round, remarking that he recollected sleeping on the floor of the hall and seeing the stars shining through the glass roof by night during the riots. It appeared that he was one of a large guard of students who were ordered out by Dr. Whewell of Trinity to defend the place. At Liverpool a busy trade was unearthed ; some casks labelled " Bitter Salts " were opened on the quay, and thirty-three dead bodies were found ready for transport to Edinburgh, the produce of Irish and English graveyards.

Investigations were made, and this supply was checked. At last the body-snatchers took to worse courses still. Burke and Hare in Edinburgh began to murder people in 1827 to sell their bodies to the anatomists. Their method was to suffocate them by a pitch plaster, or by their hands tightly pressed over the nose and mouth after they had been rendered helpless by intoxication. The criminals were finally detected and convicted, Burke confessing to thirty-three murders. The public excitement was intense, and another murder was found in London. Parliament was at last aroused to the necessity of some change, and passed an Act giving to the anatomical schools the bodies of unclaimed persons dying in institutions and of those whose friends made no objection. But for a long period the public terror continued, and the resurrectionist was the most real

and dreaded ghost of the time.   Before artificial
teeth were a success, the tooth collector was another
horror.   He hunted around the battlefields of the
Peninsula and graveyards at home, tearing healthy
teeth from the corpses, from which he made huge
gains.

6. ANATOMY, PHYSIOLOGY, AND PATHOLOGY

The real glory of the time, the work which
distinguishes it from other ages, is the astonishing
growth of physical and applied science.   It was
the development of these subsidiary and funda-
mental studies, especially chemistry, physics, minute
anatomy, physiology, and pathology, which has
given such a different equipment to the surgeon
of the modern period.   It was during the first half
of the nineteenth century that they reached a stage
when they began to be directly helpful to the
surgeon in his daily work.

Anatomy tended to grow in two directions: first
towards histology, applied anatomy, and pathology;
and secondly towards comparative studies such as
embryology and morphology, which in turn paved
the way for the discoveries of Huxley, Darwin, and
the biologists.

In France Bichat as early as 1802 carried
anatomists into new fields, concentrating their
attention on the tissues of the body and the less

well known organs; while Magendie, Flourens,
Poiseulle, and later on Claude Bernard, devised
experimental methods of research in physiology.
Bernard became one of the greatest teachers in
Europe, discovering glycogen, and giving to his
contemporaries the first idea of internal secretions
and vasomotor activity.   The first part of Pasteur's
work comes into this period, but most of his
memorable studies on fermentations and micro-
organisms are later.

In Britain the discoveries of Sir Charles Bell on
the nervous system, which led to the distinction
between sensory and motor nerves, the knowledge
of the work of the facial nerve, and Bell's nerve
itself; of Marshall Hall in 1833 on the reflex action
of the spine and medulla; Waller's studies of
nerves; and W. B. Carpenter's general physiology,
represent important advances.   We can point also
to substantial progress in surgical anatomy by
Abraham Colles, by Cooper, Liston, and Syme, and
the discoveries of Bowman on the eye, the kidneys,
and on striated muscle.

But even these studies were overshadowed for
the time by the absorbing interest shown in pathology; whether or no it was a result of Hunter's
influence, much of the best work of the time was
directed to the analysis of the effects of disease on
the tissues, until at times detractors said that the

chief aim of the surgeon and physician seemed
to be a knowledge of the results of diseases rather
than its prevention or cure. This was especially
the case in the new Vienna School, where men
like Skoda openly held that their work was diagnosis
only, and treatment practically impossible.

In these subsidiary sciences Germany, leaving
the realms of theory and philosophy for the first
time, attained to pre-eminence. For she produced
an extraordinary group of teachers and students
who carried all before them in physiology and
histology. The science had been placed on a firm
basis by the English physiologists of the seventeenth
century, but now, with the help of modern scientific
methods, the Germans quickly raised it to unexpected heights. One of the earliest and ablest of
these men was the anatomist, Johann Müller, the
originator and editor of *Müller's Archiv*, and a prolific discoverer. To him is due the law of specific
nerve energy, the recognition of the lymph hearts
in the frog, of Müller's duct, and numerous other
details. He was the great inspirer and trainer
of many pupils, such as Theodore Schwann, who
demonstrated the axis cylinders of nerves, the
action of the yeast plant in causing fermentation,
and, not least, the identity of the cellular structures
in animal and vegetable tissues.

Among Müller's other pupils were J. Henle, the

anatomist and histologist, to whom we owe our knowledge of the kidney tubules and the different varieties of epithelia ; von Kolliker, the comparative anatomist and embryologist ; and, above all, von Helmholtz, who, among many other achievements, showed the universality of the law of the conversion of energy, measured the velocity of the nervous impulse, and proved that the muscles are the main source of animal heat. He finally devoted himself to mathematical physics, where he ranks next to Lord Kelvin as one of the greatest thinkers of the age ; and, finally, Du Bois Reymond, who worked out the electrical phenomena of the muscle nerve preparation and discovered electrotonus. The Webers found out the inhibitory power of the vagus and analyzed the sensations, leaving us the so-called Weber's law. We must pass over such great discoverers as Purkinje and Remak in this long list, and merely mention Hyrtl of Vienna as the most popular teacher of anatomy in this period.

Von Liebig in 1826 began at Giessen those investigations into organic chemistry which have led to such immense results at the present time, rendering possible not only agricultural chemistry, but also the study of metabolism in the body.

The most stimulating of all these teachers in anatomy, physiology, and the allied sciences was, perhaps, Carl Ludwig, inspiring as he did so much of the investigations of subsequent times. He himself devoted prolonged study to the theory of the circulation. Even by 1850 it was clear that many of the greatest advances in these sciences were due to this group of Germans, weighty as the English and French contributions were.

7. Conclusion

We have now come to the end of our survey of the early history of surgery in Britain. This has been extended beyond its originally prescribed limit to include the last great renaissance of science preparatory to the modern period.

One cannot but be impressed by the extent to which the progress of the art has been influenced by periods of scientific enthusiasm, of humanitarian effort, of military needs, as well as by different forms of organization and by the advent of men of special genius. Thus the rise of universities and hospitals in the twelfth century, the military and gild organization later on, the officially regulated training of Tudor times, the new growth of science in the seventeenth century; and, again, private initiative and effort, as seen in the formation of voluntary hospitals and hospital and other schools in the eighteenth century, with the outburst of scientific investigation at the end of it, have all borne their fruits. It is open for discussion whether the advances were greater under socialistic regulation by the State and gilds, or under individualism, competition, and private effort. And if we narrow the question by agreeing that State licensing and examination is always desirable for the protection of the public, it would still be debatable which of these systems has given us the greatest progress in the surgical art and the best form of education.

AUTHORITIES AND BOOKS OF REFERENCE

J. FREIND : A History of Physick.
RASHDALL : Universities of Europe, vols. i. and ii.
JOH. H. BAAS : Outlines of the History of Medicine.
ANTONY A'WOOD : Athenæ Oxonienses, vol. i., f. 257; ii., f. 71-85.
  History of the City of Oxford. Ed. Andrew Clark.
SIR J. CLIFFORD ALLBUTT : Historical Relations of Medicine and Surgery to the end of the Sixteenth Century. 1905.
  Service and Mediæval Thought. Harveian Lecture, 1900.
SIR C. A. CAMERON : History of the Royal College of Surgeons in Ireland. 1886.
W. RIVINGTON : The Medical Profession in the United Kingdom. 1888.
E. T. WITHINGTON : Medical History from the Earliest Times. 1894.
ALEX. DUNCAN : Monuments of the Royal Faculty of Physicians and Surgeons, Glasgow.
THE Grace Books of the University of Cambridge. Delta ed. by Miss Bateson, and Gamma ed. by Dr. J. Venn.
J. FLINT SOUTH : Memorials of the Craft of Surgery in England.
F. H. GARRISON : Introduction to the History of Medicine. 1913.
SIR D'ARCY POWER : The Elizabethan Revival of Surgery.
  How Surgery became a Profession in London.
  Notes on Early Portraits of Banister and Harvey. Proceedings Royal Society of Medicine, vol. vi., 1912.
EDINBURGH Medical Journal: Scott Moncrieff, December, 1912; Finlay, March, 1865; J. Gairdner, February, 1867.
A COLLECTION of Royal Grants and Other Documents Relative to the Constitution and Privileges of the Royal College of Surgeons of Edinburgh, from 1505 to 1813.
JOHNSON : History of St. Peter's Hospital in Bristol.
HEARNE : Annales de Trokelowe (Oxford Edwardian Code), p. 347.

Ch. Singer: Thirteenth Century Miniatures.   Proceedings Royal
Society of Medicine, vol. ix., 1918.

John of Arderne: On Fistula, etc.   Ed. D'Arcy Power.   Early
English Text Society, 1910.

Journal of the Royal Army Medical Corps, vols. xiv.-xxii.

J. F. Malgaine : Essai sur l'Histoire de la Chirurgie.

Rotuli Hugonis de Welles, 1209-1258.

Wickersheimer: La Médicine et les Médicins a l'époque de la
Renaissance.

John S. Billings: A History of Surgery, contained in vol. i. of
Dennis's System of Surgery.   1895.

National Dictionary of Biography.

H. C. Burdett: Hospitals and Asylums of the World, vol. iii.,
p. 49.

Ashley : Introduction to the Economic History of England.

G. Unwin: Guilds and Companies of the City of London.
Industrial Organization in the Sixteenth and Seventeenth
Centuries.

Le Roulx: Les Hospitalliers.

W. Porter: The Knights of Malta.   1883.

Fincham : The Order of St. John of Jerusalem.

J. Venn: Early Collegiate Life.
The Works and Life of J. Caius.

Mostyn Reid: The Errand of Mercy.

Corpus Jur., Can. : Decretals, Gregory IX., lib. iii., t. 50, cap. 9.
Gregory IX., lib. v., t. 12, cap. 19.

J. Rae : Deaths of the Kings of England.

E. G. O'Donoghue : The Story of Bethlehem Hospital.

Morris : History of the London Hospital.

W. Munk : Roll of the Royal College of Physicians.

Cooper: Annals of Cambridge, vol. i., pp. 263-323.

Gunning : Customs and Ceremonies of the University of Cambridge, p. 141.

Historical MSS. Commission Reports.

The Bodleian Quarterly Record, vol. i., No. 1.

The New Statesman, April, 1917, Supplements on Professional
Associations.

Michael Foster : Lectures on History of Physiology, 1901.

Alex. Macalister : A Lecture on History of Study of Anatomy
in Cambridge, 1891.

Dr. J. F. Payne: Harveian Lecture.   B. M. J., vol. i., p. 200,
1896.
Fitzpatrick Lecture.   B. M. J., June 27, 1903.
        „   „   B. M. J., vol. ii., p. 1353, 1904.

Sir Norman Moore: History of St. Bartholomew's Hospital, 1919.

History of the Study of Clinical Medicine in the British Isles.

Fitzpatrick Lecture, 1905.

         „   „   1906.

Schola Salernitana, 1908.

The Progress of Medicine at St. Bartholomew's.

R. M. Clay : Mediæval Hospitals of England.

Bransby B. Cooper: The Life of Sir Astley P. Cooper.

S. Paget : The Life of John Hunter.

The Life of Ambroise Paré.

Albert H. Buck: The Growth of Medicine from the Earliest Times.

J. J. Walsh : Medieval Medicine.

Bailey: Medical Institutions of London.   B. M. J., June, 1895.

J. Hingston Fox: J. Fothergill and His Friends.

J. Munro Smith: History of the Royal Infirmary, Bristol.

Fuller: History of the University of Cambridge.

Rotuli Parliamentorum, vol. iv., pp. 130, 138, Parliament IX., Henry V.

Robert Hare: MS. Records in Registrary of University of Cambridge.

Statutes of University of Oxford, codified, 1636. Ed. J. Griffiths.

Register of University of Oxford by Boase. Ed. Andrew Clark.

Foster : Alumni Oxonienses.

Royal College of Surgeons of England Calendar (Text of Charters and Historical Summary).

Peter Lowe : Whole Course of Surgery, 1597.

Gale: Institution of a Chirurgeon, 1563, and an Excellent Treatise on Wounds.

Hall : Select Observations on English Bodies.

Cooke: Mellificium or Marrow of Surgery.

Supplementum Mellificii.

R. Wiseman : Eight Chirurgical Treatises.

Woodall : Surgeons' Mate, 1612,

The Viaticum, 1617.

Alex. Read : The Manual of Anatomy.   1638.

A Treatise on the First Part of Surgery, 1634 and 1638.

Harvey : Anatomical Exercise on the Motion of the Heart and Blood in Animals.   1628.

Ch. Whytte : A Noble Work of Surgery, 1532.

J. Halle : Chirurgia Parva Lanfranci.

A Very Fruitful and Brief Work on Anatomy.

VICARY: A Profitable Treatise on the Anatomy of Man (Early English Text Society). Ed. Furnival.

CLOWES: Proved Practice for Young Surgeons.

SIDNEY YOUNG: Annals of the Barber Surgeons of London. 1890.

MACLEAN: Dissolution of Chantries. Bristol and Gloucester Archæological Society, Trans., vol. viii.

EPISCOPAL Visitations—*e.g.*, Norwich, 1594; Gloucester, 1612, 1634, 1640, 1741.

YORK: Barber Surgeons Ordinary (Early English Text Society). Full Text York Archives, and Dr. Auden's MSS.

BRISTOL: Latimer: Annals of Bristol.
Little Red Book, 1395, 1418, 1439.
Ordinances of the Barber Surgeons, 1652, MSS.
Burgess Rolls and Chamberlain's Accounts, and Braikenbridge MSS.

NEWCASTLE: D. Embleton on Barber Surgeons, Arch. Æliana, vol. xv., p. 229.
Ordinances of the Barber Surgeons at Society of Antiquaries, Newcastle.
Brand's History of Newcastle, and MSS; in possession of the existing company of Barber Surgeons.

THE Gloucester Journal, July 30, 1728.

EXETER: Rose-Trump: Kalendars and Trade Gilds. Transs of Devons. Assoc., 1912.
Hoker: Commonplace Book, p. 323.

E. BAIN: Merchant and Craft Gilds of Aberdeen.

NORWICH: W. Rye, Calendar of Freemen, 1285-1600.
Ci Williams: Barber Surgeons of Norwich.
   ,,   List of Masters of Barber Surgeons.
   ,,   Ordinances of Barber Surgeons. See the Antiquary, 1900.

TOULMIN SMITH: English Gilds.

BRENTANO: English Gilds.

OXFORD: Records of Mediæval Oxford. Ed. by Rev. H. E. Salter, 1912 (transcript of Barber Surgeons Ordinances).
Address to the Barber Surgeons of Oxford, 3rd edition, 1749.
Twynne's Collectanea, vol. iv., p. 126.
Twynne and Langbarne, vol. iv., p. 2.

RECORD Office MSS., Chancery Miscellanea, 38-46, 1387; Ordinances of London, Lincoln, and Norwich.

CHESTER: F. Simpson, City Guilds (Barber Surgeons).
Corporation Records.

Bury St. Edmunds : Tyman's Medical History of, in Proceedings of Suffolk Institute of Archæology, vols. i. and xii.

Ipswich : Great Court Book.

Southampton : Court Leet Records, vol. i., p. 146.
    J. S. Davies, History of.

Hull : J. M. Lambert, Two Thousand Years of Gild Life.

Durham : Surtees' History of.

Reading : Ditchfield, Guilds of, in the Antiquary, vol. iv., p. 141.

Worcester : Corporation Records.

Salisbury : C. Haskins, Ancient Trade Guilds and Companies of. 1912.

ANNALS

850. Hotel Dieu.

800–1250. Salerno.

1048. First Hospital of St. John of Jerusalem.

1050. Hospital at Monte Cassino.

1086. Nigel, military surgeon.

1113. Knights Hospitallers.

c. 1100. Albucasis died.
Beginning of leprosy epidemic and of separation of medicine and surgery.

1123. St. Bartholomew's Hospital Charter.

1139. Third Lateran Council.

1150. Barber Surgeons in Germany.

1163. Council of Tours.

1180. Buckland Brewer Priory for Nursing Sisters.

1180. Roger of Parma.

c. 1200. Rise of universities, hospitals, and craft gilds.

1201–77. Salicet, William.

1205–95. Theodoric.

1207. St. Thomas's Hospital burnt.

1224. Imperial Decree on Surgery.

1234. Decretal, Gregory IX. on Surgery.

1247. Bethlehem Priory.

1252. Richard of Wendover, Anatomist.

1254. Examinations at St. Côme.

1260–1320. Henri de Mondeville.

1260. Bologna Medical School.

1299. Edward I. corps of military surgeons.

c. 1300. Bernard Gordon, Gilbertus Anglicanus.

1302. Magister Rogerus, cirurgicus at Oxford.

1308. London B.S. Gild recognized.

1310. Council of Bezières.

1316. Mundinus' *Anatomy.*

1345. York B.S. sent to Bruce.

1348. Oxford B.S. Gild.

1349. The Black Death.

1350. London B.S. lectures.

1363. Guy de Chauliac's *Surgery.*
Statute. All craftsmen to join gilds.

1369. Military Surgeons Gild.
Lincoln B.S.

c. 1370. Hospitals at York, Canterbury, Preston, Bridport, mentioned.
Statute. Apprenticeship for seven years.

1376. John of Arderne's *On Sinuses.*

1380. Mirfield's *Breviarium.*

1387. Inquisition as to rules of gilds.
London B.S. Hall, existing.

1398. Cambridge statutes on medical study.

1395. Bristol B.S. ordinances.

1400. York B.S. ordinances.

1415. Morstead at Agincourt.
London B.S. powers confirmed by the city.

1421. Law regulating practice in England.

1423. London Academy of Medicine.

1435. Ordinances of military surgeons.

1436. *Statute.* Gild ordinances require sanction of magistrates.
1446. Dublin B.S. charter.
1462. London B.S. charter.
1470. Ambulances of Isabella.
1493. The Composition of London surgeons.
1497. Jerome of Brunswick.

1505. Edinburgh B.S. incorporated.
Aberdeen University opened.
Cambridge licences for surgery.
1511. *Statute.* Episcopal licences.
1514. Vigo's *Practica Copiosa.*
1518. Royal College of Physicians.
1529. London B.S. revised ordinances.
1540. *Statute.* London surgeons and B.S. united.
1541. Caius lecturing in Cambridge.
1542. *Statute* exempting herbalists.
1543. Vesalius' *De Fabricâ.*
1544. St. Bartholomew's revived.
1545. Paré on shot wounds.
1547. Religious trusts of gilds seized.
Bethlem Hospital revived.
1551. Maggi on shot wounds.
1555. York B.S. anatomy lectures.
1556. Oxford and Cambridge Edwardian Statutes.
1563. Gale's *Handbook.*
Statutes. Apprentices and monopolies regulated.
1565. Halle and Clowes, writings of.
1567. Edinburgh B.S. exemption from juries.
1572. Dublin B.S. charter and union of surgeons.
1581. Banister's lectures.
Lumleian lectures.
1592. Edinburgh University founded.
Death of Ambroise Paré.
1599. Glasgow Royal Faculty.

1601. Poor law of Elizabeth.
1604. *Statute.* London B.S. new rules.

1612. Woodall's *Surgeon's Mate.*
1614. York B.S. lectures.
1617. Apothecaries' charter.
1624. Oxford Reader in Anatomy.
Surgeons impressed for war.
1628. Harvey's *Exercitatio.*
1629. London B.S. new charter.
1636. Oxford Laudian statutes.
Glisson, Regius Professor at Cambridge.
1638. Read's *Anatomy.*
1643. Gale's lectures.
1652. Wiseman at Worcester fight.
Bristol B.S. new ordinances.
1655. Regimental surgeons.
1662. Royal Society founded.
Students at St. Bartholomew's.
1690. Physicians' Dispensary.
1695. Students at St. Thomas's.
Edinburgh Corporation of Surgeons and Apothecaries.
1696. St. Peter's Hospital, Bristol.
1698. Arris' lectures.

1712. Dublin University Medical School.
1715. Westminster Dispensary.
1718. Edinburgh, separation of barbers and surgeons.
1719. Glasgow separation.
Westminster Hospital.
1720. Edinburgh, Monro's lectures began.
Cheselden lectures at St. Thomas's.
1725. Guy's Hospital.
1726. Edinburgh Medical Degrees.
1728. Dublin, Jervis Street Hospital.
1729. Edinburgh Royal Infirmary.
1734. St. George's Hospital.
1736-7. First Provincial Hospitals, Winchester and Bristol.
1787. Edinburgh Royal Medical Society.

1740. London Hospital.
1742. Pringle, Sir John, Surgeon-General.
1745. London B.S. separated.
      Company of Surgeons of London.
      Middlesex Hospital.
1748. The Hunters at Windmill Street.
1752. *Statute.* Murderers anatomized.
1756. John Hunter at St. George's.
1765. Pott's lectures at St. Bartholomew's.
1769. Guy's Hospital lectures.
1773. Medical Society of London.
1778. Edinburgh Royal College of Surgeons.
1784. Dublin Royal College of Surgeons.
1787. Abernethy's lectures at St. Bartholomew's.
1793. Death of Hunter.

1800. Royal College of Surgeons in London.
      Sir A. Cooper's lectures at Guy's.
      Brodie and Baillie at Windmill Street.
      Nitrous oxide tested by Beddoes.
1804. Charles Bell comes to London.

1805. Royal Medical and Chirurgical Society.
1813. Hunterian Museum opened.
1814. Abraham Colles, *On Fractures.*
1815. Apothecaries' Act.
1827. The Burke and Hare murders began.
1828. University College Hospital.
      Medical Schools at Birmingham, Bristol, and Sheffield.
1832. Anatomy Act.
      British Medical Association.
1833. J. Syme's lectures at Edinburgh.
1834. Liverpool Medical School.
      Poor Law Amendment Act.
      R. Liston at University College, London.
1836. Registration of births and deaths.
1840. Fergusson at King's College Hospital.
1843. Royal College of Surgeons of England.
      Hypnotism used by Elliotson.
1844. Nitrous oxide used by Wells.
1844-6. Ether used successfully by Morton.
1846. Semmelweiss, puerperal fever.
1847. Chloroform used by Simpson.
1855. Garcia's laryngoscope.
1858. Medical Registration Act.

INDEX

202

PRINTED IN GREAT BRITAIN BY BILLING AND SONS, LTD., GUILDFORD.